Living with Grief: Spirituality and End-of-Life Care

Edited by
Kenneth J. Doka & Amy S. Tucci
Foreword by Keith G. Meador

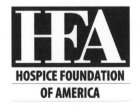

HOSPICE FOUNDATION
OF AMERICA

This book is part of Hospice Foundation of America's *Living with Grief* series.

This book is part of HFA's *Living with Grief*® series.

Ordering information:

Call Hospice Foundation of America: 800-854-3402

Or write:
Hospice Foundation of America
1710 Rhode Island Avenue, NW #400
Washington, DC 20036

Or visit HFA's Web site:
www.hospicefoundation.org

Assistant Editor: Keith Johnson
Layout and Design: The YGS Group

Publisher's Cataloging-in-Publication
(Provided by Quality Books, Inc.)

Living with grief : spirituality and end-of-life care /
    edited by Kenneth J. Doka & Amy S. Tucci ; foreword by
    Keith G. Meador.
        p. cm.
    Includes bibliographical references and index.
    LCCN 2011920483
    ISBN-13: 978-1-893349-12-4
    ISBN-10: 1-893349-12-8

    1. Bereavement--Religious aspects. 2. Terminal care
--Religious aspects. 3. Spiritual life.   I. Doka,
Kenneth J. II. Tucci, Amy S. III. Hospice Foundation
of America.

BL65.B47L54 2011   204'.42
                               QBI11-600014

Dedication

For Leah Siegel
(1966-2010)

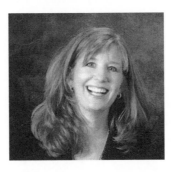

Extraordinary mother to Teagan, Wyatt, and Oliver; loving wife of Eric Loehr; caring sister to Michael Siegel; and the dynamic and devoted daughter of Hospice Foundation of America (HFA) Board Member Myra MacPherson, who was the wife of the late Jack Gordon, chairman of HFA for many years.

Leah was an accomplished producer for ESPN and a three time Emmy Award winner. She was diagnosed with metastatic lobular carcinoma, a form of breast cancer, days after the birth of her third child. Throughout two years of illness, she found meaning in her own life, enriched the lives of those around her, as well as the lives of strangers, with her wise and witty blog, which was read by 45,000 visitors. She left an inspiring and lasting legacy for her children.

She, too, came to live out loud.

Contents

Foreword

Keith G. Meador

Spiritual care at the end of life is fundamentally about hope and Berlinger and Jennings succinctly and thoughtfully engage this issue in their chapter of this volume saying, "Hope is not mere optimism." The profundity and significance of this statement cannot be overstated in our contemporary therapeutic culture (Shuman & Meador, 2003) with its proclivities to embrace such movements as "positive psychology" and the myriad of self-help efforts, which mean well but frequently end up offering some version of mere optimism rather than substantive hope. The substantive hope that those suffering and dying among us yearn for calls for a textured and robust response to suffering characterized by awareness of the past, cognizance of the current context, and a vision of the possible within the particularities of a life story. These particularities, embodied over a lifetime and narrated by the communities which have claimed us, give rise to that which gives substance to our hope. This hope is qualitatively different from that which is commonly offered by a culture captive to "optimistic" illusions of cure and promises of palliation, while frequently indulging in an avoidance of the soulful depths and contextualized complexities of the lived journeys of those who suffer. There is good reason that we often avoid these soulful depths. As Arthur Frank has said, "One of our most difficult duties as human beings is to listen to the voices of those who suffer" (1995, p. 25). But, if we can get past our fear of hearing these voices as they challenge the seductive illusions of our therapeutic culture and engage them—willing to honor the spiritual depths of those who suffer in the fullness of their particular stories—perhaps we can provide spiritual care with an integrity that bears witness to a hope that is much more than "mere optimism" and will sustain its central role in hospice care as a purveyor of hope and human flourishing even into death.

While fully acknowledging the very significant work of pain management and "doing something" that has been part of the modern hospice movement since its founding by Dame Cicely Saunders, the highlighting of spiritual care offered by this volume reminds us of the strong challenge embodied by Saunders to, at times, be simply intentionally present with the suffering and dying, thereby honoring the depths of human fullness and flourishing as individuals and as members of communities, even when dying. The important role of those who are suffering and dying in teaching all of us how to live the examined life well within an awareness of our own mortality is a crucial, and frequently unappreciated, part of rightly understanding the significance of spirituality and spiritual care at the end of life. Norman Wirzba offers a paradigm for considering the very real hope offered to all of us by those who are dying when he states that, "When we learn to accept and bear our pain together, we develop the habits that best equip us to build communities that acknowledge and celebrate our need for each other. When we fully and without rivalry welcome others, even those who seemingly do not have much to offer in return, we recognize our interdependence and learn the arts of sharing, forgiveness and gratitude" (2006, p. 86). The dying can easily seem to have little to offer in return to those surrounding them and caring for them unless we who are healthy today truly appreciate our interdependence with those who are dying while appreciating our own inevitable mortality.

The inextricable interdependence of our health as articulated by Wendell Berry when he comments that, "Health is not just the sense of completeness in ourselves but also is the sense of belonging to others and to our place; it is an unconscious awareness of community, of having in common" (1995, p. 90) is just as applicable to our understandings of death if rightly considered. How a community narrates and interprets suffering and death is frequently formed by spiritual, religious, and faith understandings, albeit with increasing diversity of faith traditions represented within the formation of such understandings for both individuals and the communities they constitute. Much effort in recent years has gone into attempts to split the notions of *religion* or *faith traditions* and *spirituality*, which has had limited success and has frequently appropriated intellectually naive public-private dichotomies that have limited credible utility. I have no interest in perpetuating such dichotomies and would appeal to an understanding of a spirituality and spiritual care that has most frequently been formed and/or informed by some amalgamation of faith traditions and practices that can be discerned if we commit to know the person for whom we give care in the fullest sense of their personhood. In this context of genuine discernment, the possibility of finding authentically hopeful meaning and redemptive potential in the face of suffering and death seems most feasible. Dying and grieving people seek to find meaning and redemptive understandings of their story with both being frequently elusive. Good spiritual care will allow others to join them on that journey, seeking a substantive and formed hope without apology, but likewise without any presumption of easy answers along the way.

Jonathan Lear, a philosopher and psychoanalyst at the University of Chicago, has given us a frame for considering "radical hope" in the face of cultural devastation and loss through the lens of the response of the visionary leader of the Crow people, Plenty Coups, when confronted with a substantial loss of many of his people and their land. Lear provides a way of envisioning a substantive and transforming hope in the face of such a devastating loss that could easily leave a person and community in despair. His embrace of the "prophetic dream" within his Native American spiritual tradition gives insight into ways of narrating the appropriation of historically interpreted faith traditions into substantive hope within diverse spiritual traditions. Lear argues that, "Plenty Coups's hope is manifest in his fidelity to his prophetic dream.... The dream was a manifestation of radical hope.... If we can make the case that this stance was a manifestation of courage, we could presumably come to see how radical hope can be not just psychologically advantageous but a legitimate response to a world catastrophe" (Lear, 2006, p. 115). Plenty Coups's negotiation of what represented a cataclysmic loss for the Crow people—through his spiritual maturity and wisdom embedded in a resilient hope of substance and vision—gives us a lens through which to conceive of a rich engagement of a hope formed by a textured and robust spirituality as we consider spiritual care of the suffering, dying, and grieving among us.

Keith G. Meador, MD, ThM, MPH, is the Vice Chair for Faculty Affairs, Professor of Psychiatry and Professor of Preventive Medicine, and Professor, Center for Biomedical Ethics and Society, at Vanderbilt University. Dr. Meador previously established and directed centers at Duke University's Medical Center and Divinity School, focusing on the intersections of religion and health. His scholarship builds on his clinical, research, and teaching background in mental health, practical theology, and public health, seeking a better understanding of the interaction of individual and socio-cultural contributors to health and human flourishing. He also directs the national initiative, Mental Health and Chaplaincy, for the Department of Veterans Affairs.

REFERENCES

Berry, W. (1995). *Another turn of the crank*. Washington, DC: Counterpoint.

Frank, A. (1995). *The wounded storyteller: Body, illness and ethics*. Chicago: University of Chicago Press.

Lear, J. (2006). *Radical hope: Ethics in the face of cultural devastation.* Cambridge, MA: Harvard University Press.

Shuman, J, & Meador, K. (2003). *Heal thyself: Spirituality, medicine, and the distortion of Christianity.* New York: Oxford University Press.

Wirzba, N. (2006). *Living the Sabbath: Discovering the rhythms of rest and delight.* Grand Rapids, MI: Brazos Press.

Acknowledgments

We always enjoy writing the acknowledgments. It is an incredible accomplishment that the Hospice Foundation of America (HFA) can produce a book annually as part of the annual *Living with Grief*® event while upholding the organization's mission and goals. Even more amazing is that this is managed by a miniscule staff that includes Spence Levine, Lisa McGahey Veglahn, Sophie Viteri Berman, Kristen Baker, Susan Belsinger, Marcia Eaker, Krista Renenger, Marceline Bateky, Lindsey Currin, and Karyn Walsh. This gives us one more opportunity to thank them and a supportive Board of Directors for all their efforts. Naturally, we also are indebted to and wish to thank the 2011 authors, who made this book a reality by submitting excellent chapters under tight deadlines. Finally, we wish to recognize the continuing legacy of the late Jack Gordon, former chair of HFA, who began the *Living with Grief*® series and whose dreams for HFA live on today.

It is so often the case, as we learn from this book, that hospice and palliative care is ahead of much of medicine's curve. Unlike most medical care practiced in the United States today, hospice and palliative care providers consider the whole person, which includes a person's spiritual side. On behalf of HFA, I want to acknowledge hospice and palliative care teams that recognize the importance of spirituality. Whether individuals come from the Southern Baptist, Catholic, Jewish, or Buddhist (or other) faith traditions, whether they believe in a higher power or have another belief system, whether they are atheist or agnostic, their spiritual nature is often a critical part of their lives and deaths and is valued and cared for by hospice and palliative care providers.

I would also like to acknowledge my co-editor Ken Doka, who this year in particular, was the perfect co-editor. As an ordained Lutheran minister, a member of the National Consensus Conference on spiritual palliative care, and an internationally-recognized expert on death, grief, and bereavement, Ken provided the knowledge and skills that make this book a significant contribution to the field. Hopefully, its readers will include not only those who already embrace the concept of spirituality as an element of patient care, but also those who have yet to incorporate spiritual care into their practices.

—Amy S. Tucci

As always, it is wonderful to work with Amy. She continues to offer solid editorial skills, deep insight, and a strong commitment to hospice and palliative care. This book would not be possible without her constant oversight.

There are so many family and friends that I need to thank. My son and daughter-in-law, Michael and Angelina, and my grandchildren, Kenny and Lucy, not only provide love, but also insist that I balance my life—always a challenge. In addition, I want to acknowledge Kathy Dillon, my Godchildren—James and Austin Rainbolt, Scott Carlson, Christine Romano, Dylan Rieger, and Keith Whitehead—and their families, especially Keith's new bride Adria, as well as my sister, Dorothy, my brother, Franky (and all of their families), and friends Eric Schwarz, Lynn Miller, Larry Laterza, Ellie Andersen, Jim, Karen, Greg Cassa, Linda and Russell Tellier, Jill Boyer, Tom and Lorraine Carlson. Good neighbors including Paul Kimbal, Carol Ford, Allen and Gail Greenstein, Jim and Mary Millar, Robert and Tracey Levy, Fred and Lisa Amore, and Chris and Dorotta Fields watch over my house when I travel and me when I am home.

Colleagues at the College of New Rochelle, the Association of Death Education and Counseling (ADEC), and The International Work Group on Death, Dying, and Bereavement (IWG) offer stimulation and friendship. I also thank The College of New Rochelle President Stephen Sweeny, President-Elect Judith Huntington, Vice-President Dorothy Escribano, Dean Marie Ribarich and Program Director Wendi Vescio, and Faculty Secretaries Diane Lewis and Vera Mezzaucella for their ongoing encouragement and support.

—Kenneth J. Doka

Spirituality and End-of-life Care

One of the most significant and enduring contributions of hospice care is the concept that effective medical care—and not just at the end of life—must be holistic. Life-threatening illness is not just a medical problem, but also a psychological, social, familial, economic, and spiritual difficulty. While life-threatening illness encompasses all of these dimensions, it is only recently that significant attention has been placed on the spiritual aspects. Emerging research has emphasized that illness: evokes a series of spiritual reactions such as anger at God or moral guilt (Doka, 2009); is a major way that persons cope with illness (Siegel & Schrimshaw, 2002); provides a mechanism for offering support (Siegel & Schrimshaw, 2002; Townsend, Kladder, & Mulligan, 2002); and influences end-of-life decisions (Koenig, 2004; Phelps et al., 2009). In fact, research even indicates that a physician's own spiritual values may affect the options and information offered to patients (Seale, 2010). It is even suggested that spiritual and religious beliefs may have physiological benefits such as lowering blood pressure or enhancing immune function, though here the research has shown some inconsistency (Dane, 2000; Sephton, Koopman, Shaal, Thoresen, & Spiegel, 2001; Miller & Thoresen, 2003; Lin & Bauer-Wu, 2003; Olive, 2004; Stefanek, McDonald, & Hess, 2005).

Yet while religion and spirituality are critical concepts, they are difficult to define. For some scholars, including the author of our foreword, Dr. Keith G. Meador, there is little distinction between *religion* and *spirituality.* Here, spirituality is simply seen as a manifestation of a radical individualism that emphasizes personal uniqueness while ignoring the collective quality of shared religious beliefs or seeks to de-institutionalize religious identity (Bregman, 2006).

For others, though, the distinction is a useful one: recognizing the inherent personal nature of an individual's beliefs even if they do draw from the shared beliefs of a recognized faith community. The International Workgroup on Death, Dying and Bereavement defines spirituality as being "concerned with the transcendental, inspirational, and existential way to live one's life" (1990, p. 75). The Consensus Conference, a national meeting of scholars in this area, agreed to the following definition of spirituality:

> Spirituality is the aspect of humanity that refers to the ways that individuals seek and express meaning and purpose and the way they experience their connectedness to the moment, to self, to others, to nature, and to the significant or the sacred. (Puchalski, et al., 2009, p. 887)

Naturally, such a definition expresses the most common factors—that is, such a definition is by nature a statement of what everyone can accept. Miller's definition is more poetic:

> Spirituality relates to our souls. It involves the deep inner essence of who we are. It is an openness to the possibility that the soul within each of us is somehow related to the soul of all that is. Spirituality is what happens to us that is so memorable that we cannot forget it, and yet we find it hard to talk about because words fail to describe it. Spirituality is the act of looking for meaning in the very deepest sense; and looking for it in a way that is most authentically ours. (1994)

To Miller, spirituality is inherently individual, personal, and eclectic. Miller also connects his definition to religious beliefs that often frame an individual's spirituality. Religion, however, is more collective. Religion is a belief shared within a group of people. Miller again offers a lyrical perspective:

> Now religion works in a very different way. While spirituality is very personal, religion is more communal. In fact, if you take the words back to its origins, "religion means that which binds together," "that which ties things into a package." Religion has to do with collecting and consolidating and unifying. Religion says, "Here are special words that are meant to be passed on. Take them to heart." Religion says, "Here is a set of beliefs that form a coherent whole. Take them as your own." Religion says, "Here are people for you to revere and historical events for you to recall. Remember them." Religion says, "Here is a way for you to act when you come together as a group, and here's a way to behave when you're apart". (1994)

Such a distinction emphasizes the individual nature of spirituality. It acknowledges the influence of religion while reaffirming that, however important, religious affiliations alone are not likely to be the sole determinant of spiritual beliefs. Often developmental outlooks, personal experiences, and cultural perspectives will join with religious beliefs in shaping an individual's spirituality.

The chapters in this first section both reaffirm and explore the role of religion and spirituality in end-of-life care and offer strategies and techniques for allowing patients and families to utilize effectively their spirituality as they cope with life-threatening illness. Thrane and Ferrell begin this section with an excellent overview of the role of spirituality and religion at life's end. They stress that suffering is inherently spiritual as it often involves a component of finding meaning in one's life and death. One of the most important aspects of their chapter notes that while spirituality can facilitate adjustment to illness and mortality, it can complicate as well. Spiritual beliefs can sometimes be a source of distress for patients and families. In Murray's case, the patient struggles with a belief that both he and his wife are damned and face an eternity of suffering. In other situations, there may be incongruous beliefs that complicate the dying process or subsequent grief. In *A Grief Observed,* for example, C. S. Lewis (1963) wrestles with the seeming contradiction between God's power and mercy as he watches his wife die a painful death. Others may suffer needlessly, viewing palliative care as thwarting God's will or holding unrealistic hope for a miracle.

Doka furthers this discussion of spirituality by exploring the ways that spirituality changes through the life cycle. To Doka, spiritual development is a lifelong process that begins as soon as one is able to search for meaning. Doka also emphasizes that spiritual development is inherently related to our developing understanding of mortality. As we become closer to our own terminality, three spiritual needs become paramount: to have lived a meaningful life, to die an appropriate death, and to find hope beyond the grave.

All the chapters emphasize the need for spiritual assessment as an integral aspect of patient care. The Consensus Conference (Puchalski, et al., 2009) recommended that all patients undergo a spiritual screening—that is, a quick determination as to whether patients (and intimate network) are experiencing serious spiritual issues. Those that are having such difficulties should be referred to a board-certified chaplain for a full spiritual assessment. The Consensus Conference also suggested that spiritual history should be included in the general history of the patient. Puchalski reviews one of her pioneer methods of assessing spirituality, her FICA analysis (faith, importance, community, address). As Puchalski notes, this is one of many methods, some of which she also reviews. It should be understood that the use of standardized instruments such as FICA should be a tool to engage in serious spiritual dialog rather than an **end** in itself. Spiritual assessments should be done even when the patient is comatose or has dementia because such assessments can assist surrogates in making end-of-life decisions. Moreover, since spiritual issues continue to change at the end of life, spirituality needs to be continually reassessed.

Berlinger and Jennings reflect on the ways that religious and spiritual beliefs may influence the ways that individuals who are dying and their surrogates approach ethical dilemmas at the end of life. Their excellent overview of the range of conflicts that can result underlies two other key issues. The first is that surrogates may not necessarily share the same values and beliefs as the patient. Helping clarify these potential conflicts through spiritual assessment can facilitate decision-making. Such clarification should respect the surrogate and family's spiritual values as well as the patient's. In an earlier piece, Jennings (2008) called for a more social ecological approach to ethical decision-making—that is, to move away from a totally individualistic orientation toward ethical decision-making by realizing the effects of such decisions on the surrogate and the intimate network of family and friends. This leads to the second point. These ethical decisions affect not only patients and their intimate networks, but also medical professionals. Such professionals have their own values and beliefs and can experience moral distress when there are disparities between their choices and beliefs and those of the patient and family (Doka, 1994).

Assessment empowers intervention. The next two chapters offer tools for intervention. Baird addresses the role of ritual. Before history, there was ritual. Prehistoric graves offer mute testimony to the rituals that accompanied the end of life. Rituals are liminal; they speak to us on both a conscious and unconscious level. Baird's chapter reviews the many times and ways that ritual offers a powerful intervention before and after death.

Fink offers another set of interventive tools. As one of the critical spiritual needs is to have lived a meaningful life, legacy work can affirm that one's life truly mattered. Fink offers a number of tools: dignity therapy, life review, reminiscence, and ethical wills. We might add to this list living eulogies, where family and friends share their memories and stories while the patient is still alive, reminding them of the connections and contributions the patient has made to others. Naturally, legacy work requires sensitivity. Some individuals may have led highly destructive lives, leaving a legacy of broken relationships. Should legacy work be undertaken here—and there remains a choice not to do so—it may focus on the lessons learned that the client would wish to pass on to others.

The last two chapters in this section address spiritual care from an organizational perspective. Piotrowski describes a trans-disciplinary approach to spiritual care. By that, Piotrowski advocates for a multidisciplinary team approach that addresses, in a holistic manner, the medical, social, psychological, spiritual, and financial needs of the patient and family. Some hospices emphasize the role of spirituality by beginning team meetings with a chaplain-led discussion of the hopes and dreams of the client instead of the traditional introduction that would focus on the patient's disease and symptoms.

Fife describes a model program, VITAS, to provide effective spiritual care. Fife notes the critical role of organizational commitment and ongoing training and describes the five spiritual needs that are central to that commitment. Interestingly enough, Fife reaffirms that pain control is an essential prerequisite to spiritual care—reinforcing the holistic model of care that is Dame Cicely Saunders', the founder of hospice, most enduring legacy.

REFERENCES

Bregman, L. (2006). Spirituality: A glowing and useful term in search of a meaning. *Omega: The Journal of Death and Dying, 53*(1/2), 5–26.

Dane, B. (2000). Thai women: Mediation as a way to cope with AIDS. *Journal of Religion and Health, 38*, 5–21.

Doka, K. J. (1994). Caregiver distress: If it so ethical, why does feel so bad? *Critical Issues in Clinical Care Nursing, 5*, 346–347.

Doka, K. J. (2009). *Counseling individuals with life-threatening illness.* New York: Springer.

Jennings, B. (2008). Death at an early age: Ethical issues in pediatric palliative care. In K. Doka & A. Tucci (Eds.), *Living with grief: Children and adolescents* (pp. 99–119). Washington, DC: Hospice Foundation of America.

Koenig, H. (2004). Religion, spirituality, and medicine: Research findings and implications for clinical practice. *Southern Medical Journal, 97*, 1194–1200.

Lewis, C. S. (1963). *A grief observed*. New York: Bantam.

Lin, H., & Bauer-Wu, S. (2003). Psycho-spiritual well being in patients with advanced cancer: An integrative review of the literature. *Journal of Advanced Nursing, 44*, 69–90.

Miller, J. (1994, November). "The transforming power of spirituality." Presentation to a conference on transformative grief, Burnsville, NC.

Miller, W., & Thoresen, C. (2003). Spirituality, religion, and health: An emerging research field. *American Psychologist, 58*, 1–19.

Olive, K. (2004). Religion and spirituality: Important psychosocial variables frequently ignored in clinical research. *Southern Medical Journal, 97*, 1152–1153.

Phelps, A. C., Maciejewski, P. K., Nilsson, M., Balboni, T. A., Wright, A. A., Paulk, M. E.,…Prigerson, H. G. (2009). Religious coping and the use of intensive life-prolonging care near death in patients with advanced cancer. *Journal of the American Medical Association, 301*(11), 1140–1147.

Puchalski, C., Ferrell, B., Virani, R., Otis-Green, S., Baird, P., Bull, J.,… Sulmasy, D. (2009). Improving the quality of spiritual care as a dimension of palliative care: The report of the Consensus Conference. *Journal of Palliative Medicine, 12*, 885–904.

Seale, C. (2010). The role of doctors' religious faith and ethnicity in taking ethically controversial decisions during end-of-life care. *Journal of Medical Ethics, 36*, 677–682. doi:10.1136/jme.2010.036194

Sephton, S., Koopman, C., Shaal, M., Thoresen, C., & Spiegel, D. (2001). Spiritual expression and immune status in women with metastatic cancer: An exploratory study. *Breast Journal, 7*, 345–353.

Siegel, K., & Schrimshaw, E. (2002). The perceived benefits of religious and spiritual coping among older adults living with HIV/AIDS. *Journal for the Scientific Study of Religion, 41*, 91–102.

Stefanek, M., McDonald, P., & Hess, S. (2005). Religion, spirituality and cancer: Current status and methodological challenges. *Psycho-Oncology, 14*, 450–463.

Townsend, M., Kladder, V., & Mulligan, T. (2002). Systematic review of clinical trials examining the effects of religion on health. *Southern Medical Journal, 95*, 1429–1434.

CHAPTER 1

Spirituality, Religion, and End-of-Life Care

Betty Ferrell and Susan Thrane

In 2009, a National Consensus Conference was convened to address the need to improve spiritual care within palliative care. The conference was born from the growing awareness that most settings of care fail to provide optimal spiritual care to those with serious illness and those at the end of life. One of the outcomes of the conference was development of a consensus definition of spirituality: "Spirituality is the aspect of humanity that refers to the way individuals seek and express meaning and purpose and the way they experience their connectedness to the moment, to self, to others, to nature, and to the significant or sacred" (Puchalski et al., 2009, p. 887). This definition captures the essence of spirituality as a broad, inclusive concept that includes the sacred but is not limited to the religious realm. Pesut wrote that "to be human is to be spiritual" (2008, p. 98), capturing the important reminder that all patients and family members are spiritual beings. There is a growing attention to spirituality as an aspect of health care, due in large part to hospice as a model of whole-person care.

Is there a difference between religion and spirituality? Some say yes and some no. Imagine the concept of spirituality in relation to canned green beans. When one looks for canned green beans in the supermarket there are several different brand names and also the store generic brand. The concept of spirituality is like thinking about all the green beans on the shelf, an all-encompassing concept that includes most forms of religion, those that may believe in a higher power but do not participate in a brand of religion, and those that find meaning in relationships or nature. Religion is more of a brand name: a label and a system of beliefs. A person can be Catholic, Protestant, Muslim, Buddhist, Hindu, or one of the many religious models in practice.

Marler and Hadaway (2002) compared several studies of spirituality versus religiosity from 1990 through 2001 and found that while the majority of Americans think of themselves as either religious or religious and spiritual, between 14% and 30% of Americans view themselves as spiritual only. Analyzing five studies that asked very similar questions, the percentage was even higher, revealing a weighted average of 73% of Americans who say they are either religious only or religious and spiritual, 18% who say they are spiritual only, and 9% who say they are neither religious nor spiritual (Marler & Hadaway, 2002, p. 292). Using four of the five studies that asked similar questions and broke the data down by age, the data are even more interesting. Of respondents age 75 and older, 78% were either religious only or religious and spiritual and 15% were spiritual only, while among adults less than 40 years old, only 63% were religious only or religious and spiritual and 23% spiritual only (Marler & Hadaway, 2002, Table 2, p. 293). Although Americans are still religion-oriented, there may be a trend away from organized religion and toward self-styled spirituality.

RELIGION

While many equate spirituality and religion, they are not the same. One definition of religion is "an organized system of beliefs, rituals, and practices with which an individual identifies and associates and includes a relationship with a Divine being" (Puchalski & Ferrell, 2010, p. 22). Religion is therefore an organized practice of spirituality. Stranahan (2008) defines religion with an important addition. She says "Religion organizes beliefs and expresses them in doctrine, dogma, rituals, symbols, and practices that are designed to foster a relationship or closeness with the sacred...*and to foster a relationship with others in the community* [emphasis added]" (p. 494).

Within any given religion there are divisions and sects. Within any sect it is possible that each gathering of adherents practice their religion or spirituality slightly differently from another group. Each person within a group likely understands or thinks of the Divine or sacred in a slightly different fashion than the person next to them. The point being, each person in the universe sees the sacred in a different way. Regardless of religious practices, spirituality is unique to each individual.

WHAT ARE THE COMPONENTS OF SPIRITUALITY?

After an extensive literature search, Vachon, Fillion, and Achille (2009) found 71 articles that revealed 11 themes in the search for a definition of spirituality. The most often cited definitions included a search for meaning and purpose; transcendence involving self or a higher being; a feeling of community or communion with self, nature, higher being, or interpersonal relationships; faith or belief system that may involve a higher being; hope; appreciation; and self-reflection. After review of these concepts, the authors suggest that spirituality is ever-evolving and involves conscious thought from within the self and that a spiritual shift may be triggered by important life events (Vachon, et al., 2009). In Clarke's article on the search for meaning as it relates to spirituality, she emphasizes that meaning must be found in a deep sense, not on the surface or merely pleasurable (2006). Meaning may be found within the self without the structure of a religion, but it should be centered on the profound and core values.

In a qualitative study of 28 patients with cancer and family caregivers, Taylor (2003) found seven categories of spiritual needs including:

- to have a relationship with a higher being;
- to be positive, show gratitude, and have hope;
- to give and receive love;
- to review spiritual beliefs;
- to create meaning and find purpose in life;
- to attend to religious needs such as prayer, participation in religious rituals, and reading spiritual texts; and
- to prepare for death in ways such as asking forgiveness, completing personal business, and finding purpose in death.

Secular contemporary music often contains spiritual references. This poignant song by George Strait illustrates the idea that in the midst of daily life, one can find the sacred in nature:

> Just walked down the street to the coffee shop.
> Had to take a break.
> I'd been by her side for 18 hours straight.
> Saw a flower growin' in the middle of the sidewalk,
> Pushin' up through the concrete
> Like it was planted right there for me to see.
> The flashin' lights,
> The honkin' horns,
> All seemed to fade away
> In the shadow of that hospital at 5:08.
> I saw God today. (Clawson, Criswell, & Kirby, 2008)

HOW DOES SPIRITUALITY FIT INTO PALLIATIVE CARE?

The 2004 release of national guidelines for quality palliative care (National Consensus Project, 2004) was a key testament to the importance of spirituality within palliative care. These guidelines identify eight domains of quality

TABLE 1. The Domains of Quality Palliative Care and Influence of Spirituality Across Domains

National Consensus Project (2009) Domains	Influence of Spirituality on Each Domain
1. Structure and Processes of Care	This domain refers to the interdisciplinary plan of care. The plan of care should address all aspects of care from all eight domains and all healthcare disciplines.
2. Physical Aspects of Care	Management of pain and other distressing symptoms may include complementary therapies. Prayer is one of the most used complementary therapies.
3. Psychological and Psychiatric Aspects of Care	Spirituality or what brings meaning to the patient and family are particularly important during the grieving process.
4. Social Aspects of Care	Spirituality may play a large part in a patient's social structure. A spiritual community may be a helpful resource for the patient.
5. Spiritual, Religious, and Existential Aspects of Care	These domains can affect care both positively and negatively. Careful and ongoing assessment are essential.
6. Cultural Aspects of Care	Spirituality is influenced by culture and vice versa. Culturally and spiritually appropriate care need to be provided to everyone.
7. Care of the Imminently Dying Patient	Spirituality is very important to patients and families at the time of death. Religious and spiritual rituals and ceremonies are key to patient and family well-being.
8. Ethical and Legal Aspects of Care	Hospitals are legally required to address spirituality. Ethical considerations of beneficence, autonomy, and non-maleficence apply to spirituality.

palliative care, one of which is spiritual care. Table 1 lists the domains of palliative care and the influence of spirituality on each domain. The National Consensus Project's guidelines and recommendations from the Spirituality Consensus Conference offer many recommendations for clinicians (Puchalski, et al., 2009). Key recommendations include making spiritual assessment standard practice for all patients with identified needs integrated into the interdisciplinary plan of care. The guidelines also propose major quality improvement efforts to create systems of care wherein attention to spiritual needs is well integrated.

Spiritual care can involve a compassionate presence, a caring touch, a prayer if requested, or participation in a religious ceremony. Spiritual care can be a sharing of the self. Spiritual healing can result from being fully present for the patient, connecting with the patient on a level of deep respect for him or her as a human being (Puchalski, Lunsford, Harris, & Miller, 2006). Spiritual care can also take place without direct intervention. Healthcare providers may pray for their patients at home or outside the institution. They may give spiritual care silently to an unconscious patient or a child too young to verbalize an understanding of spiritual care. Compassionate presence or a caring touch are also common practices to offer comfort and support.

Spiritual care can be difficult even for the most experienced caregiver. It can be difficult to engage in a spiritual discussion with someone whose beliefs differ from one's own. "Patients may utilize their spiritual or religious beliefs and values as a way to understand their illness, find meaning in the midst of their suffering, find hope in the [middle] of grief, loss and distress and find inner peace" (Puchalski, et al., 2006, p. 399). The caregiver must be open to listening to the patient's reality and respect the patient's beliefs. The caregiver may ask the patient about their spiritual or religious needs and offer to call a spiritual advisor consistent with the patient's beliefs. Excellent verbal and nonverbal communication skills are very important when participating in spiritual care (Sawatzky & Pesut, 2005). Unfortunately, a lack of education and skill related to spiritual care often mean that healthcare professionals avoid talking with patients about spirituality or responding to their needs.

SPIRITUAL SUFFERING

The importance of understanding the distinctions between spirituality and religion was captured in these words: "One of the greatest barriers to spiritual... care may be a narrow understanding of spirituality that prevents us from

TABLE 2. 10 Tenets of Suffering

1	Suffering is a loss of control that creates insecurity. Suffering people often feel helpless and trapped, unable to escape their circumstances.
2	In most instances, suffering is associated with loss. The loss may be of a relationship, of some aspect of the self, or of some aspect of the physical body. The loss may be evident only in the mind of the sufferer, but it nonetheless leaves a person diminished and with a sense of brokenness.
3	Suffering is an intensely personal experience.
4	Suffering is accompanied by a range of intense emotions including sadness, anguish, fear, abandonment, despair, and a myriad other emotions.
5	Suffering can be linked deeply to recognition of one's own mortality. When threatened by serious illness, people may fear the end of life. Conversely, for others, living with serious illness may result in a yearning for death.
6	Suffering often involves asking the question "Why?" Illness or loss may be seen as untimely and undeserved. Suffering people frequently seek to find meaning and answers for that which is unknowable.
7	Suffering is often associated with separation from the world. Individuals may express intense loneliness and yearn for connection with others while also feeling intense distress about dependency on others.
8	Suffering often is accompanied by spiritual distress. Regardless of religious affiliation, individuals experiencing illness may feel a sense of hopelessness. When life is threatened, people may conduct self-evaluation of what has been lived and what remains undone. Becoming weak and vulnerable and facing mortality may cause a person to reevaluate his or her relationship with a higher being.
9	Suffering is not synonymous with pain but is closely associated with it. Physical pain is closely related to psychological, social, and spiritual distress. Pain that persists without meaning becomes suffering.
10	Suffering occurs when an individual feels voiceless. This may occur when a person is unable to give words to his or her experience or when the person's "screams" are unheard.

Note: Adapted from Ferrell & Coyle, 2008, p. 108. Copyright Oxford University Press, Inc. Used with permission.

hearing the spiritual journeys of our patients" (Sawatzky & Pesut, 2005, p. 24). Suffering is a concept closely related to spirituality and also a key element in the goals of palliative care. Suffering can exist in all four domains of quality of life: physical, psychological, social, and spiritual. Monin and Schulz (2009) also reflected on these terms stating that:

> Suffering is a holistic construct [which] includes psychological distress, such as depression and anxiety,…physical symptoms such as pain, nausea, and difficulty in breathing,…[and] has an existential/spiritual dimension that includes loss or impairment of inner harmony, of meaning and purpose of life, and of comfort and strength in religious beliefs. (p. 2)

In 2008, Ferrell and Coyle published *The Nature of Suffering and the Goals of Nursing*, based on the synthesis of their research spanning over 20 years in the area of serious illness and end-of-life care (Ferrell & Coyle, 2008). This book identified ten themes that had emerged across these studies that describe the experience of suffering from the perspective of nursing. Table 2 lists the tenets of suffering identified through these nursing studies that also have application for all professionals. These tenets of suffering also remind us of the intricate relationship of suffering and spirituality.

SPIRITUAL CARE AND PROFESSIONAL DEVELOPMENT

When discussing spiritual care and professional development, the concept of cure versus healing must be addressed. Cure relates to the body and healing relates to the whole person. In spiritual care and end-of-life care, practitioners should realize that cure is not always possible, but healing is possible.

Spiritual Care

The essence of spiritual care is contained in the word *Namasté*, a Sanskrit word which basically means "The God (divine or sacred) within me greets (or sees) the God in you." If healthcare practitioners meet each other and their patients with the assumption that everyone contains the sacred and are worthy of respect, dignity, and compassion, then spiritual care will be easier. Spiritual care involves meeting each person on a human level, wherever they are mentally, physically, and spiritually. The essential elements of spiritual care are listed in Table 3.

TABLE 3: **The Essential Elements of Spiritual Care**

Authenticity	Humanity
Kindness	Vulnerability
Compassion	Service
Respect	Honesty
Dignity	Empathy

Note: Adapted from Baird, 2010. Copyright Oxford University Press, Inc. Used with permission.

Spiritual care requires spiritual practice. Spiritual care involves slowing down, at least for a few moments, and really being present with a person. Making eye contact, seeing into the heart, and saying with presence, "I really see you as a person; you matter" (Baird, 2010). No one is perfect at spiritual care; even chaplains or other spiritual care providers struggle to meet the unique needs of each person. The key point is to enter into spiritual care with intention, compassion, and heart.

Professional Development

In order to develop a more spiritual healthcare practice, providers must first cultivate their own spirituality. Puchalski and Ferrell (2010) have three recommendations for clinicians to promote more spiritual patient interactions. Clinicians should:

- Deepen their own spiritual practice either through a religious community or through individual reflection.
- Cultivate an intentional spiritual practice surrounding patients. This may be intentional thought at the beginning or end of the day or a prayer between patients.
- Talk to other healthcare providers about spiritual topics or questions or perhaps form a regular spiritual discussion group.

It can be difficult to address spiritual issues with others if clinicians are not addressing their own spirituality. Table 4 lists further professional considerations.

TABLE 4. **Spiritually Prepared Healthcare Provider**

Personal Attributes	Compassion
	Self-awareness
	Ability to reflect on meaning of their work and contributions
	Appropriate integration of personal spirituality into professional life
	Open to personal transformation
Professional Skills	Training in spiritual care and compassionate presence
	Competence reflective of professional discipline
	Team skills and integration of multiple disciplines
	Spiritual practice that supports professional work

Note: Adapted from Puchalski & Ferrell, 2010, p. 69. Copyright by Templeton Press. Used with permission.

A last note on professional development must include self-care for the healthcare professional. Participating in spiritual care with patients does not mean becoming enmeshed with them. Professional boundaries are still very important. Developing and deepening a personal spiritual practice can help relieve stress and prevent *compassion fatigue*, a condition that can occur when clinicians take on the problems of their patients. Participating in activities that give deep meaning and concentrating on the sacred in life assists in self-care and spiritual development.

CASE EXAMPLES

Spirituality as a Source of Support and the End of Life

Mallie Jackson was an 83-year-old woman, a widower and mother of four children and seven grandchildren. Her children had each moved away but Mallie remained in her Southern community and a devout Christian. Mallie was diagnosed with Stage IV colon cancer. Her initial prognosis was poor and her children all questioned if she should undergo surgery and chemotherapy but after meeting with her preacher, Mallie opted for aggressive treatment. She described her oncologist as "the hands of God" and she told each of her children that each day was a blessing and she was "ready for her maker."

Mallie tolerated treatment much better than expected and did well for 18 months until she developed extensive lung and liver metastasis. Until this time she attended church services regularly and was well known by the hospital staff as "Mother Mallie" because she seemed to have little regard for her own illness but often offered prayers for the staff.

When Mallie's extensive metastasis was diagnosed, her minister, children, and members of her church encouraged her to "keep fighting." Their despair at the news was clearly more extreme than her own. Mallie advised that she would need a few days to pray about her decision. The following week she asked to meet with her children, all of whom were able to come. She told her minister and children that she was at peace, that God was calling and that she would like to spend her final days in the inpatient palliative care unit, resisting the offers of her children to care for her at home. Mallie was aware of the reluctance of many in the African-American community to accept hospice and she told her preacher that she wanted to "be a witness for God's grace." Mallie welcomed her decades of friends and church members, welcoming prayers, singing, and mourning. She died peacefully on the palliative care unit.

Spirituality as a Source of Distress

Martin Garcia was a 40-year-old man admitted through the Emergency Department to the ICU. He and his wife of 10 years, Amalda, were in an auto accident. Amalda died immediately as did the other driver and Martin was suspected to be responsible for the accident. Martin had a very complicated hospital course with periods of progress for his multiple fractures and internal injuries. After 3 weeks of hospitalization, Martin unfortunately developed severe infections and subsequently developed renal failure after aggressive antibiotics, thought to be attributed to his poorly controlled diabetes and hypertension. From the time of being informed that his wife had died, Martin became withdrawn and profoundly depressed. He refused visits from an ex-wife, his mother, or the hospital social worker. When asked about chaplaincy, Martin became very angry, cursed, and threatened to pull out his dialysis catheter if a chaplain visited. He also created numerous conflicts with the physicians, nurses, and other hospital staff and was eventually avoided by most of the team.

When Martin was informed of his declining renal status and increased cardiac problems, he angrily demanded that he be allowed to die, cursing the doctors for failing, insulting the staff, and then demanding to be left alone. While he had alienated most of the staff, he has developed a bond with a young nursing assistant, Phillipe, on the night shift who bathed him early each morning. Martin confided in the aide that he was raised Catholic but hates the church and has not attended mass in 20 years. He then for the first time in this 7-week ordeal cried briefly as he told the aide that he made his wife give up the church when they met and that now "not only did I kill her, but now she will burn in hell with me." The aide responded without judgment but did tell Martin that he is Catholic and has been praying for him and Martin didn't object.

As Martin's status declined, he was expected to die within a week and was moved to a step-down unit. He was seen by the palliative care team but refused involvement of the team's chaplain. On the night shift just before Martin died, Phillipe stopped by to see Martin and, recognizing that he was dying alone, asked permission to sit with him awhile. Martin held Phillipe's hand and died peacefully. The palliative care team followed up with Phillipe in the weeks ahead, expressing their thanks to Phillipe for "being Martin's priest" and helping to make a difficult situation easier.

Case Discussion
As illustrated in these cases, spirituality is an essential element in the human experience of grief and dying. In the case of Mallie, spirituality offered

tremendous support for her, her family, and her faith community as they faced her death. For Martin, religious beliefs and an absence of spirituality created great distress as he faced the end of life, his grief, and a void of meaning. Yet even in the case of Martin, the insightful presence of a nursing assistant offered some support for both the patient and staff.

CONCLUSION

Spirituality, defined in its most encompassing sense, offers opportunity for growth, meaning, and comfort at life's end. Spirituality is integral to the experience of serious illness as patients renew their lives' meaning, often reevaluate their beliefs and relationship with a higher power, and face the ultimate loss—the end of life. For family members and friends of a dying loved one, spirituality offers a means of facing loss, addressing the meaning of life, facing mortality and allows them to wrestle with their own life's meaning.

The ever emerging field of palliative care and the legacy of three decades of hospice in the United States has demonstrated that such care is by its nature, spiritual care. Across widely varied cultures, values, and religious beliefs, spirituality transcends. It is our challenge and great opportunity as healthcare providers to continue to integrate spiritual care within all realms of care.

Betty Ferrell, RN, PhD, MA, FAAN, FPCN has been in oncology nursing for 33 years and has focused her clinical expertise and research in pain management, quality of life, and palliative care. Dr. Ferrell is a professor and research scientist at the City of Hope Medical Center in Los Angeles. She is a fellow of the American Academy of Nursing and she has over 300 publications in peer-reviewed journals and texts. Dr. Ferrell is a member of the National Cancer Policy Forum and was chairperson of the National Consensus Project for Quality Palliative Care. She is the author and co-author of several books including Textbook of Palliative Nursing Care *(Oxford University Press, 2006; 3rd edition, 2010),* The Nature of Suffering and the Goals of Nursing *(Oxford University Press, 2008), and* Making Health Care Whole: Integrating Spirituality into Patient Care *(Templeton Press, 2010). Dr. Ferrell completed a master's degree in theology, ethics, and culture from Claremont Graduate University in 2007.*

Susan Thrane, RN, MSN, OCN, is a senior research specialist in the Division of Nursing Research and Education at City of Hope. Ms. Thrane has clinical oncology experience in both pediatrics and adults. She has a background in massage, energy medicine, and engineering. Her passions in nursing are palliative and end-of-life care, spirituality, and supporting patients and families using complementary and alternative medicine. With her technical background, she also likes to find new ways to use technology to improve patient care and experiences.

REFERENCES

Baird, P. (2010). Spiritual care interventions. In B. R. Ferrell, & N. Coyle (Eds.), *Oxford textbook of palliative nursing* (pp. 663–671). New York: Oxford University Press.

Clarke, J. (2006). A discussion paper about "meaning" in the nursing literature on spirituality: An interpretation of meaning as "ultimate concern" using the work of Paul Tillich. *International Journal of Nursing Studies, 43,* 915–921. DOI:10.1016/j.ijnurstu.2006.05.005

Clawson, R., Criswell, M., & Kirby, W. (2008). I saw God today [Recorded by George Strait]. On *Troubadour* [CD]. Nashville, TN: MCA Records.

Ferrell, B. R., & Coyle, N. (2008). *The nature of suffering and the goals of nursing.* New York: Oxford University Press.

Marler, P. L., & Hadaway, C. K. (2002). "Being religious" or "being spiritual" in America: A zero-sum proposition? *Journal for the Scientific Study of Religion, 41,* 289–300.

Monin, J. K., & Schulz, R. (2009). Interpersonal effects of suffering in older adult caregiving relationships. *Psychology and Aging, 24,* 681–695. DOI: 10.1037/a0016355

National Consensus Project for Quality Palliative Care (2004). Clinical practice guidelines for quality palliative care. Brooklyn, NY: Author.

National Consensus Project for Quality Palliative Care (2009). Clinical practice guidelines for quality palliative care (2nd ed.). Pittsburgh, PA: Author.

Pesut, B. (2008). A conversation on diverse perspectives of spirituality in nursing literature. *Nursing Philosophy, 9,* 98–109.

Puchalski, C. M., & Ferrell, B. R. (2010). *Making health care whole: Integrating spirituality into patient care.* West Conshohocken, PA: Templeton Press.

Puchalski, C., Ferrell, B., Virani, R., Otis-Green, S., Baird, P., Bull, J.,… Sulmasy, D. (2009). Improving the quality of spiritual care as a dimension of palliative care: The report of the Consensus Conference. *Journal of Palliative Medicine, 12,* 885–904.

Puchalski, C. M., Lunsford, B., Harris, M. J., & Miller, T. (2006). Interdisciplinary spiritual care for seriously ill and dying patients: A collaborative model. *The Cancer Journal, 12,* 398–416.

Sawatzky, R., & Pesut, B. (2005). Attributes of spiritual care in nursing practice. *Journal of Holistic Nursing, 23*(1), 19–33. DOI: 10.1177/0898010104272010

Stranahan, S. (2008). A spiritual screening tool for older adults. *Journal of Religious Health, 47,* 491–503. DOI: 10.1007/s10943-007-9156-8

Taylor, E. J. (2003). Spiritual needs of patients with cancer and family caregivers. *Cancer Nursing, 26,* 260–266.

Vachon, M., Fillion, L., Achille, M. (2009). A conceptual analysis of spirituality and the end of life. *Journal of Palliative Medicine, 12*(1), 53–59. DOI: 10.1089/jpm.2008.0189

CHAPTER 2

Spirituality, Death, Loss, and Grief: A Life Cycle Perspective

Kenneth J. Doka

"Truly I say to you, unless you turn and become like children, you will never enter the kingdom of heaven." Matthew 18:3 (RSV)

"When I was a child, I spoke like a child, I thought like a child, I reasoned like a child; when I became a man, I gave up childish ways." I Corinthians 13:11 (RSV)

These scriptures from the Christian tradition reaffirm a reality that all faiths acknowledge: Our spirituality continually changes throughout our life. Yet despite the obvious truth of such a statement and the importance that many place in spiritual beliefs and spiritual development, spirituality, until most recently, has received limited academic study within the social and psychological sciences. Almost 40 years ago, Heenan (1972) characterized the social scientific study of religion as an "empirical lacunae"—a fact just now beginning to change. This partly reflects on the generally agnostic character of the social sciences. Part of the problem also lies in the difficulty of developing an operational definition of spirituality that is distinct from religious affiliation.

While there has been more interest and research in spirituality in the past decade, comparatively little research has focused on life cycle issues. This is unfortunate. Spirituality, even at early ages, offers a vocabulary, symbolism, and approaches to meaning-making that allow individuals ways to understand and to adapt to suffering, dying, death, and grief (Champagne, 2008). In many ways, our spirituality is confirmed, challenged, or changed as we encounter these experiences on our life's journey.

This chapter explores the ways spirituality develops and changes throughout the life cycle, focusing especially on how encounters with mortality often spur us toward spiritual development. Underlying this discussion is the importance of understanding, assessing, and supporting individuals, at any age, as they use their spirituality to make meaning in the face of death.

LIFE CYCLE PERSPECTIVES: FOWLER'S STAGES OF FAITH

Such a discussion must begin with the pioneering work of James Fowler (1981). Building on the developmental work of Piaget (1965), Erikson (1950), and Kohlberg (1984), Fowler proposed a 6-stage model of spiritual or faith development. His model does not claim that the content of faith changes at each stage. Rather, the style of faith and how we value our faith changes. For Fowler, faith is a verb—a state of being—rather than a noun. Fowler defined faith similarly to how most people define spirituality, rather than adherence to a set of beliefs.

Fowler also differentiated *conversion* from *development*. Conversion refers to a radical change of our faith narrative while development emphasizes a more gradual maturing process.

Fowler did not claim that faith development was inevitable or even essential or desirable. He believed that each person could find a sense of spiritual fulfillment at whatever stage they experienced. While Fowler notes the approximate ages for each stage, he is very clear that even an adult's spirituality can be characterized by any one of the first 3 stages.

In his stage model, Fowler was also clear that these are "snapshots" of a dynamic, ever-changing process. While Fowler's model actually begins with stage 1, Kirst-Ashman and Zastrow (2004) suggested a preceding stage 0 that they theorized offers a foundation for the development of faith and trust.

- *Stage 0: Primal or Undifferentiated* (birth to age 2). While not in Fowler's model, this stage reflects the very young child's perception of his or her environmental safety. To Kirst-Ashman and Zastrow (2004), this sense of safety allows the child to develop a sense of trust that underlies the development of faith.
- *Stage 1: Intuitive-Projective* (ages 3–7). The child is just beginning to develop a sense of self and the world. Highly egocentric, the child is trying to make rudimentary sense of his or her experience. They have a difficult time differentiating between the real and the fantasized. Authority is externalized—symbolized by size or other symbols of power and position, e.g., teachers or uniforms.
- *Stage 2: Mythical-Literal* (ages 6–12). The child now exhibits concrete operational thinking. Now, children have begun to understand communal

faith stories and use them to order their experiences. They often have a strong sense of fairness and reciprocity: Good gets rewarded and evil punished. If there is a sense of a deity, it is often anthropomorphic.

- *Stage 3: Synthetic-Conventional* (adolescence). The emerging adolescent now begins to clearly identify with the beliefs of his or her community. This conformity becomes a basis of the adolescent's identity. While the adolescent conforms to these beliefs, they remain largely unexamined.

- *Stage 4: Individualistic-Reflective* (early adulthood). The young adult begins to critically examine and own his or her beliefs rather than simply adhere to the beliefs of others. Symbols, myths, and rituals are accepted if they are personally meaningful. Persons in this stage can tolerate controversy, disagreement, and questions.

- *Stage 5: Conjunctive* (midlife). In midlife, persons become aware of their own mortality. As they evaluate their life, they become conscious of their own underlying polarities: young/old, masculine/feminine, and their constructive/destructive sides. Persons are more open to accept the truths of other positions even as they hold to their own faiths.

- *Stage 6: Universalizing.* This is a stage that only a few individuals such as Mother Theresa or Gandhi may achieve. In this enlightened state, the individual can exhibit a total altruism and a sense of deep connection to all of humanity.

Fowler's model is a valued one for a number of reasons. It represents a relatively early attempt to map spiritual development. Fowler was sensitive to the dangers and limitations of such a model. Like many stage models, it often fails to fully characterize the diversity or complexity of how individuals struggle with their spirituality through the life cycle. Also, like many stage models, it lacks a clear empirical basis and it has a clear linear and prescriptive bias. Stage 6 seems a desired, even if generally unattainable, goal for spiritual development. Nonetheless, many of Fowler's ideas will be evident in the ensuing discussion.

SPIRITUALITY IN THE LIFE CYCLE

Childhood

Rather than a stage approach, it is probably more useful to begin by acknowledging the inherent relationship of spirituality to underlying themes of meaning-making, identity, and connection. In short, from the very beginning of personal consciousness, as we grapple with our place in the world and the meaning and significance of events, we inevitably encounter spiritual issues and concerns.

Naturally, this begins early in childhood. When a very young child, perhaps a little older than a toddler, asks "Why?" after picking up a dead bird, he or she is asking an inherently spiritual question. One of the difficulties of stage-based and developmental approaches is that these frameworks often focus on what the child can or cannot cognitively comprehend. In doing so, they miss an essential corollary: that children, even at young ages, are *trying* to make sense of their world.

Coles (1990), in his classic work *The Spiritual Life of Children*, employs a useful metaphor. Coles was trained as a psychiatrist by Erich Lindemann—famous for his initial work on grief (Lindemann, 1944). As Coles worked in the 1950s with children stricken with polio, he listened carefully to how the children's spirituality helped them adapt to this encounter with illness and mortality. Their spiritual stories, whether from the Bible or the Koran, helped them look not only upward but inward.

Children, Coles claims, are *spiritual pilgrims*. By that, he means that children try to make sense of the world without the cognitive-spiritual maps that adults possess. Their sense-making is a spiritual work in progress, a continued exploration in a territory they do not fully know or understand.

In that quest, they often attempt to apply the broad understandings that have been conveyed to them within their spiritual traditions. Christian children, for example, often reflected on the incarnation, taking comfort from the reality that Jesus really knew what it was like to struggle with childhood. To Islamic children, surrender to the will of Allah was a major theme while Jewish children looked to the moral precepts of their faith to guide them through life.

As children encounter illness, loss, and grief—whether their own or of someone close to them—they seek to understand the event, to make sense of their experiences. This inevitably is a spiritual process as they turn to their beliefs, faith narratives, rituals, and practices. They may not yet have the cognitive capacity to reach conclusions. Their questions may show innocence and naiveté. When her maternal grandmother died, my 3-year-old granddaughter took comfort in the belief that her grandmother would watch her from heaven. However this led to a very practical concern. Would her grandmother be able to see her on the toilet? The point is that children, no matter how young, are trying to make sense of their world and are inevitably encountering their spirituality.

Adolescence

This spiritual process continues into adolescence. In much developmental theory, adolescence is often divided into three periods. *Early adolescence* corresponds to the middle school years while *middle adolescence* is identified with high school. *Late adolescence* is harder to define but is generally recognized as the period after high school but before the child becomes psychologically (and perhaps economically) independent of his or her parents. In some cases, for example, when a child graduates high school and immediately finds a job, marries, joins military service, or establishes an apartment, the period can be quite short or even nonexistent. In other cases, such as when the child is in college, dependent on the family, or living at home, this period can be protracted.

In each of these periods, the adolescent struggles with three core issues: independence, intimacy, and identity. It is the latter process that underlies spirituality (Quinn, 2008). As part of identity, the adolescent, now capable of critical thought, asks, "What do I believe?" There is a process of differentiation here. Adolescents are aware of what they have been taught by parents, family, and spiritual leaders. The question now becomes what beliefs will become part of their personal identity—that is, what beliefs they will personally own.

Moreover, as adolescents begin to develop critical thinking, they are encountering their own spiritual questions. "Why do people suffer and die?" "Why do disasters occur?" While these questions may have been encountered earlier in their lives, there is greater depth to that reflection.

In addition, as the adolescent struggles with their individuality, there can be a growing awareness that death—nonexistence—represents a great threat to their emerging identity. In some cases, this may lead to extensive denial of death or challenges to death evident by the dangerous behaviors common in this stage of life.

The threat of death can be accentuated by the stress and isolation the adolescent experiences. With an emerging sense of individuality, a growing sense of aloneness may emerge. "There is no one like me" easily becomes "There is no one who fully understands me." These questions of meaning, identity, and aloneness are core existential, and therefore spiritual, concerns.

For some adolescents, the transition to college can deeply accelerate this process. Here, they may be exposed to new people and ideas. Professors may challenge their once pat answers. For some students, the loss of their prior beliefs can be profound, creating a sense of crises and loss that can even generate grief over their now-lost faith (Barra et al., 1993).

While adolescents may question or review their spirituality, it remains a critical aspect of adolescent stability. While research on spirituality and adolescence is limited (Petersen, 2008), studies of religiosity have found a positive correlation with an adolescent sense of well-being, positive life attitudes, altruism, resiliency, school success, health, and positive identity, as well as a negative correlation with alcohol and drug use, delinquency, depression, excessive risk-taking, and early sexual activity (Benson, Ruehlkepartain, & Rude, 2003).

Early Adulthood

Developmental theorists often stress that early adulthood focuses on externals: obtaining a job or career, developing an independent lifestyle, and possibly finding a life partner and establishing a family (Erikson, 1963). Internal issues such as spirituality often take second place to these core developmental tasks.

Such a perspective neglects the spiritual issues inherent in mate selection and child rearing. As one selects a life partner, the question of spiritual compatibility looms large. Individuals need to reflect on their own core spiritual values and determine to what degree those values need to be shared by their partner. "Does my partner need to share my faith? How will we raise our children? What spiritual values, rituals, and practices do we wish to pass on to our children? What religious holidays or events will we choose to celebrate or commemorate?" Often these questions may be re-evaluated once children actually arrive as the decisions once settled or tabled now have new currency.

Moreover, there are aspects of early adult life that do, at least in a remote way, raise the specter of mortality. As young adults begin to accumulate assets and responsibilities, they may begin to execute documents such as wills, advance directives, or guardianships. Such documents assume an implicit recognition of mortality, which inevitably invokes spirituality.

Middle Adulthood: Spirituality and the Awareness of Mortality

The growing awareness of personal mortality spurs us toward spiritual development (Doka, 1988, 1995). A number of conditions and circumstances contribute to an awareness of mortality in middle adulthood. First, as adults reach their 30s, 40s, and 50s, they begin to experience varied physiological and sensory declines that reinforce the reality of aging and eventual death. Women experience menopause and both men and women may experience a gradual diminution of sexual prowess. This, too, is a vivid reminder of loss and aging. And, as Kastenbaum and Aisenberg suggest (1976), there may be an inverse relationship between reproductive capability and a sense of terminus.

Second, there is a dramatic increase in the mortality rate for those in their 40s or older. Adults in midlife may begin to experience the death of peers from causes other than accident or suicide. The loss of others in one's cohort is a vivid reminder of personal vulnerability.

A third factor is that adults in midlife begin to see their own parents aging and dying. Not only does this create new relationships with aging parents, it reinforces one's own aging and death. Adults in midlife may also have children establishing their own families and careers, reinforcing the reality that one's own cohort is advancing in age toward distant but inescapable death. As Moss and Moss state:

> The loss of a parent represents the removal of a buffer against death. As long as the parent was alive the child could feel protected, since the parent by the rational order of things was expected to die first. Without this buffer there is a strong reminder that the child is now the older generation and cannot easily deny his or her own mortality. (1983, p. 73)

Other factors in midlife may also increase awareness of mortality. Grandparenthood is often interpreted as a mark of age. Preparation for retirement, albeit somewhat distant, reiterates the passage of time. The approach of what is perceived as a significant birthday (e.g., 40, 50) may also be understood as a mark of age. A serious operation, health crisis, or onset of chronic illness may increase the awareness of mortality.

It would seem, then, that given the differing conditions and circumstances that lead to the awareness of mortality in adults, that this awareness can develop gradually, over time, as a person slowly becomes aware of physical declines and personal vulnerability. In other cases, this awareness may be a sudden insight in response to a crisis. When any given individual achieves this recognition will vary depending on the situations and circumstances of life.

While it is beyond the scope of this chapter to fully discuss the implications of this emerging awareness of personal mortality (see Doka, 1988, 1995), one such implication is a modified sense of time. The child primarily looks toward the future. Time is measured from birth. The older person may be more oriented toward the past. The "time remaining" is considered both cogent and short. Neugarten (1972) theorizes that this restructuring of time occurs in middle age as the increasing awareness of finiteness leads one to think in terms of both time since birth and time left to live.

As the recognition of time shifts, there are profound implications for the sense of self. As stated earlier, the recognition of personal mortality leads to a reassessment of one's self-identity. The middle-aged person must consider what one has been, what one wished to be, and what one can still become. As Erikson (1963) states, generality becomes a central issue. "What is to be left behind?" "What is the legacy?"

There is some support for the idea that death anxiety peaks in midlife (see Doka, 1988, 1995; Neimeyer, 1994). Middle-aged persons, though, become aware of death when their commitments and opportunities are extensive. Death becomes the haunting specter that may yet rob them of the opportunity to achieve their goals and enjoy the fruits of their efforts. Death perhaps is the greater terror, stalking midlife, threatening goals and plans, heralding incompleteness, and even for some, suggesting the futility and meaningless of existence. We can posit that the recognition of eventual death may encourage spiritual reflection in middle adulthood. Perhaps this crisis forces midlife adults to confront life and find or construct meaning as to avoid the terror of death. Aware of limited time, even if it is measured in decades, a midlife adult becomes deeply concerned that his or her life have meaning. There is a reassessment of one's life. For those generally content with their past and present life and content with the direction life seems to be taking, this concern with meaning may not be overly troublesome. They need simply to reaffirm the meaning they have already found and perhaps recommit to their current goals. Such persons may reprioritize their goals and themes, deciding, for example, to spend more time with family. Others may wish to make major life changes or feel despair over their choices that seem too late to correct. There may simply not be enough time to find meaning in a heretofore meaningless existence. Perhaps the "midlife crisis" is a manifestation of this frantic concern to achieve meaning by rearranging one's present and future.

The awareness of mortality engenders a re-evaluation with the state of present life and triggers a renewed interest in the afterlife. As we confront our own mortality, we are likely to reflect on our beliefs and hopes about any afterlife. In short, the awareness of mortality in midlife prompts a period of spiritual reflection and reevaluation (Wink & Dillon, 2002).

Later Life

Spiritual development remains a cogent issue in later life (Wink & Dillon, 2002). Here, the recognition of mortality becomes an awareness of finitude (see Marshall, 1980). Death is perceived as closer. This does not mean that we expect to die immediately, but rather that we realize that death is part of life. Hence we are reluctant to perceive or plan too far into the future. Time is now primarily viewed through the past (Neugarten, 1972).

Both Marshall (1980) and Butler (1963) see the awareness of finitude prompting a *life review process.* Here the individual reviews his or her past life to affirm that it had meaning and value. To Erikson (1963), a successful life review means that the older person can view life with a sense of *ego integrity,* that is, a sense that one has lived a worthwhile life. Thomas and Cohen (2006) found it helpful for participants to identify their major spiritual turning points since this process facilitates meaning-making by helping identify varied spiritual interpretive frameworks. The ultimate goal of life review is, as Marshall states, that one's life should be a "good story" (1980). If the life review is not successful, one may perceive that one's life has been wasted, yielding to a sense of despair.

Much like the awareness of mortality, the timing of the development of an awareness of finitude is inexact. Events such as nursing home institutionalization, illness, or frailty can certainly accelerate it. On the other hand, a chronic illness that leads to an expectation of an early or imminent death can create an awareness of finitude and subsequent life review even in the very young (Bluebond-Langner, 1965).

The awareness of finitude also often engenders a concern with a good, appropriate death (see Marshall 1980; Weisman, 1972). This means that the person wants to die in a way consistent with their values, wishes, or earlier life. On a practical level, that might mean that older persons are intent on instructing their adult children about their estate, advance directives, and even their wishes about funerals and other rituals. Yet the discussion suggests that this may create a paradoxical situation: As older adults may need to address the issues of their death, middle-aged children struggling with their own awareness of mortality may be deeply threatened by their parents' death and hence avoid such discussion. That same paradox may trouble adult children's end-of-life decision making as they confront the death of an older parent.

As we approach life's end, the issue of beliefs in the afterlife looms larger. Lifton and Olson (1974) suggest that we look for a form of symbolic immortality. This can be found in varied religious beliefs of an afterlife or transcendence or through a more secular emphasis on a return to the cycle of life. It may also be a sense that we live on in our progeny or work and accomplishments.

It has been debated whether or not older persons become more religious as they age. Such a debate avoids the central issue: that later life raises profound spiritual concerns of meaning and connection. Whether we reconnect, review, or renew prior religious beliefs or whether we are even open to new religious experiences, we are likely to engage in some forms of spiritual searching—perhaps religious, perhaps not—but spiritual.

CONCLUSION

Naturally, the life cycle is just one factor that influences spiritual development. Other events such as caregiving experiences or life-threatening illness can also influence spiritual development (Doka, 2003–2004, 2008), as can a myriad of other factors including culture, gender, education, or social class.

Nonetheless, life cycle development should always be part of spiritual assessments. Such assessments can include identification and analysis of spiritual turning points (Thomas & Cohen, 2006) or spiritual autobiographies that trace spiritual development throughout the life cycle. The value of these techniques is that they can reveal sources of spiritual strengths and facilitate coping, connection, and meaning-making. They also reaffirm the truth of Jesuit philosopher Pierre Teilhard de Chardin's observation that "perhaps we are not human beings on a spiritual journey but spiritual beings on a human journey."

Kenneth J. Doka, PhD, MDiv, is a professor of gerontology at the Graduate School of the College of New Rochelle and senior consultant to the Hospice Foundation of America. A prolific editor and author, Dr. Doka's books include Living with Grief: Diversity and End-of-Life Care; Living with Grief: Children and Adolescents; Living with Grief: Before and After Death; Death, Dying and Bereavement: Major Themes in Health and Social Welfare; Living with Grief: Ethical Dilemmas at the End of Life; Living with Grief: Alzheimer's Disease; Men Don't Cry, Women Do: Transcending Gender Stereotypes of Grief; Living with Grief: Loss in Later Life; Disenfranchised Grief: Recognizing Hidden Sorrow; Children Mourning, Mourning Children; Death and Spirituality;

Living with Grief: After Sudden Loss; Living with Grief: When Illness is Prolonged; Living with Grief: Who We Are, How We Grieve; Living with Grief: At Work, School and Worship; Caregiving and Loss: Family Needs, Professional Responses; AIDS, Fear and Society; Aging and Developmental Disabilities; *and* Disenfranchised Grief: New Directions, Challenges, and Strategies for Practice. *In addition, Dr. Doka has published more than 60 articles and book chapters. Dr. Doka is editor of* Omega *and* Journeys: A Newsletter to Help in Bereavement.

REFERENCES

Barra, D. M., Carlson, E., Maize, M., Murphy, W., O'Neal, B., Sarver, R., & Zinner, E. S. (1993). The dark night of the spirit: Grief following a loss in religious identity. In K. Doka & J. Morgan (Eds.), *Death and spirituality* (pp. 291–308). Amityville, NY: Baywood Publishing Co.

Benson, P., Ruehlkepartain, E., & Rude, S. (2003). Spiritual development in childhood and adolescence: Toward a field of inquiry. *Applied Developmental Science, 7,* 205–213.

Bluebond-Langner, M. (1965). *The private worlds of dying children.* Princeton, NJ: Princeton University Press.

Butler, R. (1963). The life review: An interpretation of reminiscence in the aged. *Psychiatry, 26,* 65–76.

Champagne, E. (2008). Living and dying: A window on (Christian) children's spirituality. *International Journal of Spirituality, 13,* 253–263.

Coles, R. (1990). *The spiritual life of children.* Boston: Houghton Mifflin.

Doka, K. (1988). The awareness of mortality in mid-life: Implications for later life. *Gerontology Review, 1,* 19–28.

Doka, K. (1995). The awareness of mortality in mid-life: Implications for later life (revised). In J. Kauffman (Ed.), *The awareness of mortality.* Amityville, NY: Baywood.

Doka, K. (2003-2004). The spiritual gifts—and burdens—of caregiving. *Generations, 27*(4), 45–48.

Doka, K. (2008). *Counseling individuals with life-threatening illness.* New York: Springer.

Erikson, E. H. (1950). *Childhood and society.* New York: Norton.

Erikson, E. H. (1963). *Childhood and society* (2nd ed.). New York: Norton.

Fowler, J. (1981). *Stages of faith: The psychology of human development and the quest for meaning*. San Francisco: Harper & Row.

Heenan, E. (1972). Sociology of religion and the aged: The empirical lacunae. *Journal for the Scientific Study of Religion, 11*, 171–176.

Kastenbaum, R., & Aisenberg, R. (1976). *The psychology of death*. New York: Springer.

Kirst-Ashman, K., & Zastrow, C. (2004). *Understanding human behavior and the social environment* (6th ed.). Belmont, CA: Brooks/Cole.

Kohlberg, L. (1984). *The psychology of moral development*. San Francisco: Harper & Row.

Lifton, R. & Olson, E. (1974). *Living and dying*. New York: Bantam Books.

Lindemann, E. (1944). Symptomatology and management of acute grief. *American Journal of Psychiatry, 101*, 141–148.

Marshall, V. (1980). *Last chapters: A sociology of aging and dying*. Monterrey, CA: Brooks/Cole.

Moss, M., & Moss, S. (1983). The impact of parental death on middle aged children. *Omega: The Journal of Death and Dying, 14*, 65–75.

Neimeyer, R. A. (Ed.). (1994). *Death anxiety handbook: Research, instrumentation and application*. Washington, DC: Taylor & Francis.

Neugarten, B. (1972). Adaptation and the life cycle. *Counseling Psychologist, 6*, 16–20.

Petersen, A. (2008). Spiritual development in adolescence: Toward enriching theories, research and professional practice. *New Directions for Youth Development, 118*, 119–130.

Piaget, J. (1965). *The moral judgment of the child*. New York: The Free Press.

Quinn, J. (2008). Perspectives on spiritual development as part of youth development. *New Directions for Youth Development, 118*, 73–77.

Thomas, C., & Cohen, H. (2006). Understanding spiritual meaning-making with older adults. *The Journal of Theory Construction and Testing, 10*(2), 65–70.

Weisman, A. (1972). *On dying and denying: A psychiatric study of terminality.* New York: Behavioral Publications.

Wink, F., & Dillon, M. (2002). Spiritual development across the adult life course: Findings from a longitudinal study. *Journal of Adult Development, 9,* 79–94.

CHAPTER 3

The Spiritual History: Listening to the Whole Story

Christina M. Puchalski

Over the last two decades, the role of spirituality in healthcare has increasing become a focus of research and education. Today, "spirituality and health" is a new field of healthcare. Why this interest? Today's healthcare systems are stressed; patients and healthcare professionals feel isolated and overwhelmed. Spirituality brings back the sense of a soul of medicine—where compassion becomes the central guiding principle of how healthcare professionals and patients interact and where meaning, healing, and wholeness become as important as technical cures and fixes.

Spiritual and religious beliefs have been shown to impact understanding of illness as well as healthcare decisions (Puchalski, 2002; Phelps et al., 2009). Each person has a story with spirituality being an essential part of the story. Charon (2001) describes the importance of giving space to patients' stories as a way to help them heal. By telling their story, patients can find what gives their lives meaning. This is especially true of people in the midst of suffering, stress, and illness.

Spirituality is that part of the patient's story that describes their sense of ultimate meaning and purpose. What are their sources of hope and who or what do they feel connected to? Spirituality is broader than religion. In the National Consensus Conference on Inter-professional Spiritual Care in Palliative Care (Puchalski et al., 2009), the consensus definition of spirituality is:

> Spirituality is the aspect of humanity that refers to the way individuals seek and express meaning and purpose and the way they experience their connectedness to the moment, to self, to others, to nature, and to the significant or sacred.

With this definition, spirituality is highlighted as an ongoing process; people not only find meaning but seek meaning throughout their lives and continue to express it in different ways. Spirituality also involves a sense of connectedness to the sacred, however people understand it.

SPIRITUALITY IN THE CLINICAL SETTING

Clinical settings today are very impersonal. Healthcare professionals are rushed and patients are overwhelmed. Insurance regulations, time constraints, economic realities, and complexity of treatment choices have stressed the healthcare system. These factors have overshadowed the basic tenets of what health care was founded on: service and compassion and the need to respect and value the dignity of all patients, families, and caregivers. These tenets underscore the importance of the healthcare professional relationship. It is all about the relationship—a relationship that is built upon mutual compassion and respect. Spirituality is the foundation of such a relationship-centered model. It speaks to the call to serve that all healthcare professionals share and to the sacred nature of all healing relationships. Rachel Naomi Remen writes, "The spirit is part of our daily lives as health professionals.... When we become fully present,...we open a doorway of meaning and possibility for our patients and for ourselves as well" (Puchalski & Ferrell, 2010, pp. xii–xiv). To create a whole healthcare system we must integrate spirituality fully and recognize that patients have spiritual as well as physical and psychosocial needs.

Patients and families also note the need for a more holistic approach. In numerous surveys, the majority of patients want to have their spiritual needs addressed by their healthcare professionals. For example, McCord et al. (2004) reported that patients in a family practice setting again felt that it was important for physicians and healthcare providers to address their spiritual issues and beliefs. In this study, 95% of patients wanted their spiritual beliefs addressed in the case of serious illness, 86% when admitted to a hospital, and 60% during a routine history. Interestingly, integrating spirituality into care also improves patient satisfaction with care (Astrow, Wexler, Texeira, Kai He, & Sulmasy, 2007).

Religious and spiritual themes arise often in the clinical setting. Illness can trigger many spiritual issues and therefore the clinical setting may be the first place where these spiritual issues arise. Spiritual or religious issues may be a source of support for patients or they may lead to conflict, guilt, and despair. It is important to allow patients and families to talk about these issues. Koenig and colleagues found that positive religious coping was associated with better mental health while negative religious coping was associated with poorer physical health, worse quality of life, and greater depression in medically ill hospitalized older adults (Koenig, Pargament, & Nielson, 1998). Spirituality, more broadly defined, has also been shown to impact healthcare outcomes. In one study, patients with HIV found a greater will to live and had more optimism if they also scored high on a spirituality scale (Cotton et al., 2006). Studies such as these underscore the importance of integrating spirituality more fully into patient care.

SPIRITUAL MODELS OF CARE

In the National Consensus Conference (NCC) sponsored by the Archstone Foundation and co-led by Puchalski and Ferrell, a novel model of inter-professional spiritual care was developed (Puchalski et al., 2009). In this model, every healthcare professional has the obligation to attend to patients' spiritual needs and concerns. This means that spiritual distress needs to be attended to with the same intensity as physical distress. The NCC developed specific recommendations and ways to do this. These recommendations included doing a spiritual screening or history, diagnosing spiritual distress, locating spiritual resources, and integrating these resources or distress into the treatment plan. Board-certified chaplains are recognized as the experts in spiritual care and the professionals that can work with others on the interdisciplinary team to attend to patients' spiritual concerns or help alleviate patients' spiritual suffering.

The NCC model and recommendations also address some of the reasons for the resistance to addressing spirituality in the clinical setting, including lack of time, lack of a clear definition of spirituality, or inappropriate clinician behavior such as proselytizing (Sloane et al., 2000) or lack of training. These recommendations include using validated tools for screening, history, and assessment, adhering to appropriate ethical guidelines including no proselytizing, and providing models for training of interdisciplinary health professionals. Spirituality is also described as a part of the professional and personal development of health professionals and the basis for the practice of compassion.

COMMUNICATION ABOUT SPIRITUAL ISSUES

Communication with patients and families about spiritual issues ranges from identification of spiritual issues to formal assessment (Lo et al., 2002; Puchalski & Romer, 2000). These include identifying spiritual themes and patient resources, diagnosing spiritual distress if present, and then integrating these into a treatment or care plan and making the appropriate referrals or taking another appropriate action (e.g., continued presence with patients).

During the clinical encounter, one should listen for expressions of spiritual distress and then follow up. Some of the spiritual distress diagnoses that can be identified include despair, hopelessness, abandonment by God or others, isolation from a religious community, inability to forgive, and lack of meaning. For example, a patient may say, "I have no meaning" or "What is the purpose of my life?" Or, patients may express a sense of hopelessness or despair in their conversations and behavior. Once a spiritual issue is identified, the clinician needs to consider how to treat that issue. For example, if a patient identifies a desire to seek a closer relationship to God or transcendence, the clinician can consider referring him or her to a spiritual director. The clinician could consider referral to a therapist or meaning-oriented group therapy for patients who express a sense of meaninglessness (Breitbart, 2003). Patients may express interest in yoga, meditation, or a religious ritual. Clinicians do not need to be experts in all spiritual or religious beliefs and practices; they can learn from their patients about what is important them. Clinicians can be aware of resources in their community, such as a pastoral care department in a hospital or a community yoga center, where they can refer patients for further information.

A spiritual history, screening, or assessment is a more formal part of the medical history in which the patient or family is asked about their spiritual and religious beliefs. In general, nonchaplain clinicians do a spiritual screening or a spiritual history; chaplains do a spiritual assessment. Spiritual screening or triage is a quick determination of whether a person is experiencing a serious spiritual crisis and therefore needs an immediate referral to a professional chaplain. Spiritual screening helps identify which patients may benefit from an in-depth spiritual assessment by a professional chaplain. Spiritual history-taking is the process of interviewing a patient about their spiritual beliefs and how those beliefs might impact their health care. The spiritual history questions are usually asked in the context of a comprehensive examination by the clinician who is primarily responsible for providing direct care or referrals to specialists such as professional chaplains. Spiritual assessment refers to a more extensive assessment done by board-certified chaplains that is based on a narrative process. This assessment includes a spiritual care plan with expected outcomes and plans for follow-up (VandeCreek & Lucas, 2001).

All patients should have their spiritual issues addressed in the context of their care. Chaplains are the spiritual care specialists while other clinicians function as generalists in spiritual care. Thus, all clinicians recognize and address spiritual issues with patients; they also should refer to chaplains for more intense assessment and treatment as needed.

FIGURE 1. FICA: A Spiritual History, *Puchalski, 1996*

F—Faith and Belief I—Importance C—Community A—Address in Care or Action		
F	"Do you consider yourself spiritual or religious?" - or - "Do you have spiritual beliefs that help you cope with stress (contextualize to the situation, e.g., with what you are going through right now, with dying, with dealing with pain)?"	Sometimes patients respond with answers such as family, career, or nature. Patients who respond "yes" to the spiritual question should also be asked about meaning.
I	"What importance does your faith or belief have in your life? Have your beliefs influenced how you take care of yourself in this illness? What role do your beliefs play in regaining your health?"	These questions can help lead into questions about advance directives and proxies who can represent the patient's beliefs and values. One can also ask about spiritual practices and rituals that might be important to people.
C	"Are you part of a spiritual or religious community? Is this of support to you and how? Is there a group of people you really love or who are important to you?"	Communities such as churches, temples, and mosques, or a group of like-minded friends can serve as strong support systems for some patients.
A	"How would you like me, your healthcare provider, to address these issues in your healthcare?", or ask the patient "What action steps do you need to take in your spiritual journey?"	Often it is not necessary to ask this question but to think about what spiritual issues need to be addressed in the treatment plan. Examples include referral to chaplains, pastoral counselors, spiritual directors, journaling, and music or art therapy. Sometimes the plan may be simply to listen and support the person in his or her journey.

SPIRITUAL HISTORY TOOLS

For nonchaplain healthcare professionals, the spiritual history can be integrated into the intake history, usually as part of the social history. A spiritual history is as important as any other part of the clinical history. When doing a clinical history, clinicians target specific areas. Simply listening to themes alone will not elicit all the information needed to provide good medical care. Thus, specific questions need to be asked to target areas of information regarding social support, sexuality, domestic violence, smoking, and alcohol or drug use. A spiritual history is simply a set of targeted questions aimed at inviting patients to share their spiritual and religious beliefs, if desired, and guiding them to share what gives meaning to their lives, particularly as it relates to the clinical setting, e.g., new diagnosis, loss, or other life stress.

FIGURE 2. SPIRIT: Taking a Spiritual History, *Maugans TA, 1997*

S	Spiritual belief system	Do you have a formal religious affiliation? Can you describe this? Do you have a spiritual life that is important to you? What is your clearest sense of the meaning of your life at this time?
P	Personal spirituality	Describe the beliefs and practices of your religion that you personally accept. Describe those beliefs and practices that you do not accept or follow. In what ways is your spirituality/religion meaningful for you? How is your spirituality/religion important to you in daily life?
I	Integration with a spiritual community	Do you belong to any religious or spiritual groups or communities? How do you participate in this group/community? What is your role? What importance does this group have for you? In what ways is this group a source of support for you? What type of support and help does or could this group provide for you in dealing with health issues?

R	Ritualized practices and restrictions	What specific practices do you carry out as part of your religious and spiritual life (e.g., prayer, meditation, service, etc.)?
		What lifestyle activities or practices does your religion encourage, discourage, or forbid?
		What meaning do these practices and restrictions have for you? To what extent have you followed these guidelines?
I	Implications for medical care	Are there specific elements of medical care that your religion discourages or forbids? To what extent have you followed these guidelines?
		What aspects of your religion/spirituality would you like to keep in mind as I care for you?
		What knowledge or understanding would strengthen our relationship as physician and patient?
		Are there barriers to our relationship based upon religious or spiritual issues?
		Would you like to discuss religious or spiritual implications of health care?
T	Terminal events planning	Are there particular aspects of medical care that you wish to forgo or have withheld because of your religion/spirituality?
		Are there religious or spiritual practices or rituals that you would like to have available in the hospital or at home?
		Are there religious or spiritual practices that you wish to plan for at the time of death, or following death?
		From what sources do you draw strength in order to cope with this illness?

There are several spiritual history tools that have been developed. These include FICA [see Figure 1] (Puchalski & Romer, 2000; Puchalski, 2006), SPIRIT [see Figure 2] (Maugans, 1996), and HOPE [see Figure 3]

FIGURE 3. HOPE: A Spiritual History

H	Sources of hope, strength, comfort, meaning, peace, love, and connection
O	The role of organized religion for the patient
P	Personal spirituality and practices
E	Effects on medical care and end-of-life decisions

(Anandarajah & Hight, 2001). Generally, these tools include spiritual or religious identification, what gives someone meaning, the importance of their beliefs and the way their beliefs affect healthcare decision-making, and what community affiliation, if any, they have. The FICA tool has been validated in a recent study that demonstrated that a majority of patients with cancer rated faith and belief as very important in their lives. We also showed that the FICA tool closely correlated with items from the quality of life tools assessing aspects of spirituality (Borneman, Ferrell, & Puchalski, 2010).

The spiritual history should be done as part of the routine history or can be contextualized depending on the reason for the visit. For example, if the patient is coming for a routine visit, one might address spirituality in the context of stress management or health. If the patient has just been told of a serious diagnosis, then the questions might be phrased differently. For example "Do you have spiritual beliefs that have helped you in difficult times before?"

The spiritual history is normally done during the social history section of the initial assessment as one is asking the patient about their living situation and significant relationships. The clinician can transition into how the patient cares for themselves, which includes exercise, nutrition, and then spiritual beliefs and practices or what gives one's life meaning. The spiritual history might also be taken in specific clinical situations if spiritual issues come up, for example in breaking bad news or in end-of-life situations. The spiritual history should also be taken at follow-up visits as appropriate. Figure 4 presents the spiritual history within the clinical context.

A spiritual history focuses the interview on the relationship aspect of care. It signals to the patient that the healthcare professional is interested in what truly matters to the patient and not just what is important about the illness.

Figure 4: Social History Section of an Initial Interview
(adapted from The Practice of Medicine Curriculum,
George Washington University)

Social History Section of an Initial Interview
• Important relationships; sexual history
• Occupational history
• Avocation interests
• Smoking, alcohol/drugs, seat belts, domestic violence, mood concerns
• Wellness/prevention: exercise, nutrition, spiritual beliefs

Anecdotally, medical students have often observed that "something in the room changes when I ask patients about their spiritual history." Being present can open up the possibility of what some consider to be a healing encounter. The very act of providing the patient space to share their beliefs and feelings gives him or her the opportunity to find resources of strength within themselves and possibly find ways to better cope with suffering or find inner healing. This is the basis of honoring dignity and providing respect and compassion.

Integrating Spirituality Into the Treatment/Care Plan

Once the clinician diagnoses a spiritual issue, he or she then decides how to integrate that issue into the treatment or care plan. There a several models for how to do this, developed as part of a national consensus initiative to develop spiritual care guidelines (Puchalski et al., 2009). Ideally, an interdisciplinary team of healthcare professionals that includes a board certified chaplain as the spiritual care expert develops the treatment or care plan. In settings where there is not an interdisciplinary team, such as an outpatient setting, the clinician needs to work with spiritual care professionals, e.g., outpatient chaplains, pastoral counselors, spiritual directors, community clergy, religious leaders, or culturally based healers.

The information gathered from the spiritual history needs to be documented in the patient's medical chart or electronic database. One way to do this is to follow the bio-psychosocial-spiritual model and document the assessment and plan within that holistic framework (Puchalski, 2002). An example of this is shown in the case described in Table 1 on the following page.

TABLE 1. Case Example: Bio-Psychosocial-Spiritual Model Assessment and Plan

A 68-year-old woman is dying of end-stage pancreatic cancer with well controlled pain, some anxiety, afterlife concerns, and a sense of abandonment by God.		
Dimension	**Assessment**	**Plan**
Physical	Pain is well controlled No other symptoms	Continue with current medication regimen.
Emotional	Anxiety about uncontrollable pain and discomfort when actively dying	Referral to counselor for anxiety management and exploration of issues about fear of dying. Education on how pain and other symptoms can be managed.
Social	Concerns about funeral planning, will	Refer to social worker for assistance with end-of-life planning.
Spiritual	Issues about abandonment by God, concerns about afterlife	Referral to chaplain for spiritual counseling. Continue presence and support.

(Adapted from Puchalski, 2007).

COMPASSIONATE PRESENCE

The tools described above are only guides for conversations. In a fully relationship-centered interview, the interaction stimulated by the questioning is of most value; it is not so much the answers themselves. Patients seek connection with their healthcare professionals. They want us to be fully present to them in their time of need. Also, healthcare professionals often say they feel more gratified when they can engage in profound relationships with their patients—what we have described as transformative relationships (Puchalski & Ferrell, 2010). In this model, the healthcare professional creates a sacred space for deep sharing within the clinical context. So, when asking the patient about his or her spirituality, the healthcare professional is really inviting the patient to share from their inner life, to share information that might be painful or profound. It is no less sacred than conversations at a church in the confessional or conversations whispered on a death bed to a loved love. Thus, healthcare professionals need to prepare themselves to engage with their patients at all times, but especially when patients are suffering and sharing their pain, hopes, and deepest wishes. We may utter words we pull from a tool, but we listen with an open heart in a silent space of honor.

CONCLUSION

Good medical care should be focused on the delivery of care that attends to all dimensions of a patient: mind, body, and spirit. It is the obligation of all healthcare professionals to attend to all dimensions of a patients' suffering including spiritual or existential suffering. Thus, any clinical history should have questions directed at all aspects of the patient's life, including the spiritual, particularly with the focus on identifying and treating spiritual distress. Patients' spiritual resources of strength also need to be included in a treatment plan, recognizing all the strengths patients have in dealing with stress, illness, and dying. By integrating spiritual concerns, patients may have the opportunity for healing and finding peace even in the midst of suffering or dying. All encounters with patients and families are sacred ones where space is held for support through suffering and the sharing of joy. Spirituality then forms the basis of a care system that is holistic and compassionate as it recognizes that the essential element is relationship-centered care and attention.

Christina Puchalski, MD, MS, is the executive director of the George Washington Institute for Spirituality and Health in Washington, DC, and a professor of medicine and health sciences at The George Washington University School of Medicine, where she has pioneered novel and effective educational and clinical strategies to address the spiritual concerns common in patients facing illness. Dr. Puchalski is an active clinician, board-certified in internal medicine and palliative care. Dr. Puchalski has demonstrated leadership in research and education in the integration of spiritual care across disciplines. She has received numerous awards including the Healthcare Foundation of New Jersey's Faculty Humanism in Medicine Award. She is a Fellow of the American College of Physicians and a member of Alpha Omega Alpha medical honor society. In 2009, she was awarded the 2009 George Washington University Distinguished

Alumni Award in recognition of her scholarship and leadership in spirituality, compassion, and healthcare. She has authored numerous chapters in books and edited and authored a book published by Oxford University Press titled Time for Listening and Caring: Spirituality and the Care of the Seriously Ill and Dying *with a foreword by His Holiness, The Dalai Lama. Her many publications and presentations have urged the development of a patient-centered perspective in health care, with specialization in the importance of integrating spirituality and compassion into one's professional practice. Her work has been featured on numerous print and television media including Good Morning America, ABC World News Tonight, NBC Nightly News, The Washington Post, The New York Times, and the Washington Times.*

REFERENCES

Anandarajah, G., & Hight, E. (2001). Spirituality and medical practice: Using the HOPE questions as a practical tool for spiritual assessment. [see comment]. *American Family Physician, 63*(1), 81–89.

Astrow, A. B., Wexler, A., Texeira, K., Kai He, M., & Sulmasy, D. P. (2007). Is failure to meet spiritual needs associated with cancer patients' perceptions of quality of care and their satisfaction with care? *Journal of Clinical Oncology, 25*(36), 5753–5757.

Borneman, T., Ferrell, B., & Puchalski, C. (2010). Evaluation of the FICA tool for spiritual assessment. *Journal of Pain and Symptom Management, 40*(2).

Breitbart, W. (2003). Reframing hope: Meaning-centered care for patients near the end of life. Interview by Karen S. Heller. *Journal of Palliative Medicine, 6*(6), 979–988.

Charon, R. (2001). Narrative medicine: A model for empathy, reflection, profession, and trust. *Journal of the American Medical Association, 286*(15), 1897–1902.

Cotton, S., Puchalski, C., Sherman, S., Mrus, J. M, Peterman, A. H., Feinberg, J.,...Tsevat, J. (2006). Spirituality and religion in patients with HIV/AIDS. *Journal of General Internal Medicine, 21*, 5–13.

Koenig, H. G., Pargament, K. I., & Nielson, J. (1998). Religious coping and health status in medically ill hospitalized older adults. *The Journal of Nervous and Mental Disease, 186*(9), 513–521.

Lo, B., Ruston, D., Kates, L. W., Arnold, R. M., Cohen, C. B., Faber-Langendoen, K.,…Tulsky, J. A. (2002). Discussing religious and spiritual issues at the end of life: A practical guide for physicians. *Journal of the American Medical Association, 287*(6), 749–754.

Maugans, T. A. (1996). The SPIRITual history. *Archives of Family Medicine, 5*(1), 11–16.

McCord, G., Gilchrist, V. J., Grossman, S. D., King, B. D., McCormick, K. E., Oprandi, A. M.,… Srivastava, M. (2004). Discussing spirituality with patients: A rational and ethical approach. *Annals of Family Medicine, 2*(4), 356–361.

Phelps, A. C., Maciejewski, P. K., Nilsson, M., Balboni, T. A., Wright, A. A., Paulk, M. E.,…Prigerson, H. G. (2009). Religious coping and use of intensive life-prolonging care near death in patients with advanced cancer. *Journal of the American Medical Association, 301*(11), 1140–1147.

Puchalski, C. (2002). Spirituality. In: A. Berger, R. Portenoy, & D. Weissman (Eds.). *Principles and practice of palliative care and supportive oncology* (2nd ed.) (pp. 799–812). Philadelphia: Lippincott Williams & Wilkins.

Puchalski, C. (2006). Spiritual assessment in clinical practice. *Psychiatric Annals, 36*(3), 150.

Puchalski, C. (2007). Spirituality and the care of patients at the end-of-life: An essential component of care. *Omega—Journal of Death & Dying, 56*(1), 33–46.

Puchalski, C., & Ferrell, B. (2010). *Making health care whole.* West Conshohocken: Templeton Press.

Puchalski, C., Ferrell, B., Virani, R., Otis-Green, S., Baird, P., Bull, J.,…Sulmasy, D. (2009). Improving the quality of spiritual care as a dimension of palliative care. *Journal of Palliative Medicine, 12*(10).

Puchalski, C., & Romer, A. L. (2000). Taking a spiritual history allows clinicians to understand patients more fully. *Journal of Palliative Medicine, 3*(1), 129–137.

Sloan, R. P., Bagiella, E., VandeCreek, L., Hover, M., Casalone, C., Jinpu Hirsch, T., Poulos, P. (2000). Should physicians prescribe religious activity? *New England Journal of Medicine, 342*(25), 1913–1916.

VandeCreek, L., & Lucas, A. M. (2001). *The discipline for pastoral care giving: Foundations for outcome oriented chaplaincy.* New York: Haworth Pastoral Press.

CHAPTER 4

Ethical Dilemmas and Spiritual Care Near the End of Life

Nancy Berlinger and Bruce Jennings

Q uestions about the meaning of human life, how an individual constructs a life of value and integrity, and how individuals are connected to things beyond themselves are classic philosophical questions. Persons who know they are near the end of life, or who have lived with life-threatening illness for a long time, may take a special interest in these questions. Hospice and palliative care specialists often use the terms *spirituality* or *spirituality and religion* to characterize these concerns, and are likely to characterize care offered in response to these concerns as *spiritual care*.

Spiritual care includes, but is not limited to, meeting the religious needs of a dying patient and his or her loved ones. Some healthcare professionals use the word *spirituality* to refer to a general orientation toward the nonmaterial or transcendent aspects of human life, and characterize the psychological sensibility of the person who is interested in these aspects of life as *spiritual*. The word *religion*, by contrast, implies membership in an organized community or institution built around shared beliefs, doctrines, and rituals. However, this distinction tends to break down quickly, particularly in a culture in which predominant forms of religion, Protestant Christianity in particular, emphasize a direct, personal relationship between the individual and God, thereby blurring the line between spirituality and religion, between the psychology of the individual and the sociology of the group, and between different types of experience, including private experience of transcendence and public forms of worship or communion.

Findings from qualitative studies of patients with advanced cancer suggest that most patients will characterize themselves as being spiritual, religious, or both to some extent when they are interviewed with reference to these terms, while a small minority will not identify with either of these terms (Balboni et al., 2010). This research also suggests that the word *spiritual* should not be used as a synonym for *religious*, but neither should it be used as a synonym for *nonreligious*, as some of these subjects applied both words to themselves but did not necessarily equate them. In short, in a pluralistic society, it may be impossible to capture the range of meanings and experiences associated with the terms *spirituality* and *religion*.

Ethical dilemmas that arise in the context of caring for patients whose spiritual concerns are relevant to how they wish to be cared for near the end of life often involve confusion over language, and over how to describe aspects of human experience that, by their nature, can be hard to explain. As such, it is worth remembering that data on religious affiliation is notoriously unreliable as a guide to the religious and spiritual concerns of an individual, and that a person who appears to be religiously observant may not characterize him- or herself as religious. She or he may prefer a different word, such as *traditional* or *faithful*. And while the word *spiritual* tends to have a benign or neutral connotation, some individuals find great meaning in behaviors, such as substance abuse or eating disorders, which are harmful. Therefore, spiritual values should not be assumed to be values that will be easy for a caregiver to identify and affirm.

Spiritual care, as a feature of the care of the whole person, is integral to the values of hospice, and hospice organizations offer guidance to their members on the delivery of spiritual care in hospice programs (National Hospice and Palliative Care Organization, 2001). Spiritual care is also increasingly likely to be integrated into palliative care outside of hospice settings, as board-certified chaplains, whose professional values and clinical training are already oriented toward palliative care, become more closely involved in the design and delivery of interdisciplinary palliative care in different settings.

Clergy who are not board-certified chaplains are also spiritual care providers within their congregations or other settings in which they work. Local or community clergy vary in their understanding of the spiritual needs of persons who are seriously ill or dying, their familiarity with the settings in which dying people are cared for, and their personal comfort or discomfort with end-of-life care apart from its ritual dimensions, such as saying prayers or officiating at funerals (Jacobs, 2010). Attention to the ethics of spiritual care requires healthcare institutions to consider the qualifications of those who provide spiritual care in their facility, how to differentiate between the skills needed to provide different types of spiritual care, and how to ensure that patients and loved ones are offered care that is appropriate to their needs (Robinson, Thiel, Backus, & Meyers, 2006).

ETHICAL DILEMMAS IN PROVIDING SPIRITUAL CARE

Caring for a patient near the end of life means being attentive to a whole person who, from early childhood onward, has had an inner life, a social identity, and often, a variety of identities formed in relation to different social contexts and their traditions: family, friendships, school, work, community, ethnicity, geography, religion, and others. For example, a professional who has long lived and worked on the East Coast and who self-identifies as nonreligious may continue to identify strongly with the Midwestern values of her family and with some, but not all, of the religious values with which she was raised. A dying person's spiritual life continues to evolve, and as human beings are more than representatives of cultural groups, the caregiver must be cautious about deducing a patient's current spiritual concerns from the social identity or identities that this patient, or this patient's loved ones, present to the caregiver.

Ethical dilemmas—uncertainty over how to act in a patient's best interests when the patient's wishes cannot be determined, or when all options are flawed, or when there is conflict among those involved in the patient's care, or when all of these conditions are present—may arise in the context of providing spiritual care, or with respect to values that are associated with religious beliefs and practices. Some examples of these dilemmas include:

- Situations in which caregivers are unfamiliar with the religious beliefs of a patient, how these beliefs may appropriately inform decisions about treatment and care, and how to proceed when an objection to a clinical recommendation, often concerning a decision to continue or forgo life-sustaining treatment, is framed in terms of religious belief. These situations may or may not also involve consideration of broader cultural attitudes about illness, treatment, the care of the sick, or the rights of patients, and the extent to which patients and surrogates share values.
- Situations in which a religious struggle—a belief that life-threatening illness is a test of religious faith—appears to exert undue pressure on treatment decision-making. The medical professional who must honor the informed decisions of a capacitated patient or a surrogate may wonder whether the mere presence of a religious struggle impairs decision-making capacity, or may question whether a surrogate's own religious struggle risks placing the surrogate's interests ahead of the patient's interests.
- Situations in which a patient's or surrogate's use of religious-sounding language (e.g., "miracles happen," "it's in God's hands now") leads to uncertainty on the part of medical professionals with respect to

understanding what the patient wants or what an incapacitated patient would want. The use of this language by clergy at the bedside who seek to provide comfort to a patient and loved ones but who may be unfamiliar with the medical details of a patient's diagnosis or prognosis can also contribute to communication difficulties or conflict. Medical professionals can also contribute to decision-making difficulties if they use the language of "hope" in imprecise or inconsistent ways.

- Situations in which a patient, or a surrogate for a patient who lacks decision-making capacity, makes decisions about medical care with reference to a religious or spiritual framework that excludes potentially life-saving options that could benefit the patient. Even when it is clear that a treatment refusal on religious grounds constitutes an informed refusal and a legal right, medical professionals may find such cases confusing or troubling.

The resolution or management of these ethical dilemmas requires that both healthcare professionals and healthcare institutions recognize that the values and preferences of patients concerning treatment may be related to their ongoing spiritual lives. It should also be recognized that a patient's religious beliefs (or nonbeliefs) may inform—but do not determine—their treatment-related choices. Institutions should prepare professional caregivers, as well as trained nonprofessional caregivers such as pastoral care volunteers and hospice volunteers, to recognize and respond to these dilemmas. They should invest in clinical services such as ethics consultations, conflict resolution, ethics education, and opportunities for ethical reflection on complex cases, to help caregivers resolve or manage immediate dilemmas, understand how ethical dilemmas arise, learn how to resolve conflicts, and learn how to talk with patients and loved ones about spiritual concerns that may be relevant to treatment decision-making—where ethical dilemmas typically arise.

The involvement of board-certified chaplains in all of these activities is encouraged (de Vries, Berlinger, & Cadge, 2008). Chaplains specialize in the delivery of spiritual care to seriously ill patients and their loved ones, frequently serve on ethics consultation services, and are familiar with end-of-life considerations. Board-certified chaplains are also trained for multi-faith, multi-cultural caregiving. They are likely to be familiar with the range of religious and related cultural needs that may be present in the community served by an institution providing end-of-life care. This knowledge can be extremely helpful to clinicians who are confronted by unfamiliar religious language or beliefs and may be uncertain about how to talk with patients or surrogates with reference to spiritual or religious values.

In addition to learning how to recognize and respond to ethical dilemmas as they arise in the care of individual patients, spiritual caregivers should have a well-informed understanding of the psychological dimensions of serious illness and the role of psychological factors associated with spirituality in treatment decision-making.

RELIGIOUS COPING AS A FACTOR IN TREATMENT DECISION-MAKING

Research on how patients cope with advanced cancer suggests that there is an association between a decision to use some form of life-sustaining treatment such as mechanical ventilation or cardio-pulmonary resuscitation (CPR) in the last week of life and, on the other hand, an existing practice of "positive religious coping." This means that patients whose ability to cope with serious illness is based in a belief that God works with a sick person to overcome illness may make decisions about life-sustaining treatment with reference to this belief.

This is a potentially important insight from the national "Coping with Cancer" study conducted by researchers at the Dana-Farber Cancer Institute (Phelps et al., 2009). To what extent this finding applies across patient populations is unclear. Most of the participants in this study who reported using religious coping were Christians who lived in the same geographic region of the United States. These participants were also younger, less well educated, and more likely to be uninsured than study participants who did not use religious coping. No single personal or social characteristic is likely to explain why some patients continue to choose life-sustaining interventions at the very end of life and others do not. Moreover, other research suggests that cancer patients, as a population, tend to continue other forms of potentially life-sustaining treatment, such as chemotherapy, in the last weeks of life (Harrington & Smith, 2008).

Nonetheless, a recognition that some patients or their surrogates make decisions about life-sustaining interventions with reference to values reflected in their longstanding coping practices, and that these practices can be integrally related to their religious beliefs, is essential to good communication and the support of informed decision-making near the end of life. The involvement of a mental health specialist, a social worker, or a chaplain in this discussion may be helpful in eliciting a fuller understanding of how a patient copes with illness and treatment and how past experience of coping may inform how a patient or surrogate perceives the decision at hand.

One of the reasons that this question of the role of meaning in healthcare decision-making is so difficult is that there is no neutral language available to help us talk about meaning (Geertz, 1973). Language that sounds neutral to a healthcare professional, but is derived from a particular religious tradition, may sound biased to a patient who does not identify with this tradition. In particular, healthcare professionals can fail to observe how frequently the language and structure of spiritual care is perceived as "Christian" by a patient who is not Christian. The concept of *coping* is itself associated with the field of psychology, a field that has its own interest and professional stake in questions of meaning. What a psychologist terms *coping* can also be recognized as the individual's use of familiar paradigms when faced with a challenge to one's very existence: Should one fight for life or accept death? What is the meaning of suffering and struggle? Who is in solidarity with the one who suffers? Religion is a rich source of these paradigms, conveyed through stories about how a good and faithful person confronts adversity. Confusion and conflict can arise if patients, loved ones, and professionals are not able to reconcile the moral stories that may have helped a patient weather great suffering with the epistemologically authoritative stories of medicine and science, which may seem to offer a miraculous escape from suffering (Kleinman, 1988).

Concepts such as hope and ambivalence are interwoven into these stories near the end of life, and to a discussion of them we now turn.

HOPE AS A FACTOR IN TREATMENT DECISION-MAKING

A decision to pursue medical treatment in response to the diagnosis of a life-threatening but potentially treatable condition is a decision that involves hope: the expectation that, under conditions of uncertainty, there is a reasonable possibility of a good outcome. Hoping is different from wishing. We can wish for anything and do not have to justify our wishes as reasonable. Wishing can be a method of coping with a difficult situation or expressing empathy with a person in such a situation. It can be appropriate, and welcome, for healthcare professionals to use the language of wishing: "I wish the last treatment had worked" (Quill, Arnold, & Platt, 2001).

Hope is future-oriented and directed at an object: We hope *for* something. The object of a patient's hopes may be obvious when a patient's condition is potentially curable. Patients whose conditions are chronic and progressive may also hope for specific outcomes. For some, simultaneously hoping for the best while bracing for bad news becomes a normal way of coping with the stresses of illness and caregiving, the flow of information from medical professionals, the encouraging, disappointing, or ambiguous results of treatment, and the need of the living person not to be consumed by the awareness of death.

Prognostic uncertainty does not diminish hope, but may fuel it. Hope is associated with uncertainty, and therefore with possibility, but it is not wholly dependent on clinical predictions. Research with patients with advanced cancer suggests that patients construct their sense of hope from sources that are not limited to the outcomes of treatment, and in particular, from the quality of their human relationships and their desire to continue to participate in these relationships (Smith et al., 2010). Indeed, if one is certain beyond a reasonable doubt about how things will turn out, the appropriate orientation is expectation, not hope.

Hope is not mere optimism. Encouraging a patient to "stay hopeful" or "think positive" is no substitute for clarifying whether or not it is reasonable for this patient to hope for a particular outcome. It would be unethical for a healthcare professional to encourage a patient or a surrogate to hope for something that cannot happen: for example, that a treatment will cure an incurable condition or that the use of a symptom-relieving technology will halt the progression of underlying disease. It would also be unethical to foster, or fail to correct, what amounts to a false belief—for example, that a treatment with small potential for a marginal benefit will prolong the patient's life if there is no evidence that the treatment will have any impact on the patient's overall survival—on the grounds that telling a patient the truth would cause the patient to lose hope (Smith et. al, 2010).

Clinicians face moral issues when they confront their personal psychological responses to a patient's prognosis. When successive treatments have failed to control the progression of disease but there are still treatment options with small potential for some marginal benefit, should a professional tell the patient what he or she expects will happen if a new treatment is started, based on the patient's history of response to similar interventions? Or should the professional limit him- or herself to confirming that it is still reasonable for the patient to hope that one of these options will result in tangible benefits that outweigh burdens? Is this professional conscious of how his or her own attitude toward hope may influence how he or she presents options to her patient?

Some healthcare professionals believe or have been trained that to "give hope" is part of their job or that being "hopeful," in the sense of optimistic, is a professional virtue. This belief may be strongly associated with professions such as nursing, chaplaincy, and social work and with specialties such as oncology and pediatrics, but is certainly not limited to these professions and specialties. The language of hope is also part of the language of American health care and is integral to how hospitals market themselves to prospective patients. It may also be part of a professional's own religious or spiritual life. Opportunities for ethical reflection and personal reflection offered to professionals caring for persons near the end of life should include attention to the concept and language of hope, including how individual members of different healthcare professions define hope, talk about hope, and perceive their responsibilities with respect to addressing their patients' hopes.

Adding to the complexity is that the same professionals who value giving hope, or who are in the habit of encouraging patients and loved ones to be hopeful, may be perplexed when patients or loved ones are inclined to continue treatment when a patient's condition is deteriorating no matter what interventions are attempted. These patients or loved ones may be characterized as naive or in denial, "hoping for a miracle." If these patients or loved ones are perceived to be religious, their continued hope may be (negatively) associated with their religious beliefs. Their faith is now perceived as a problem, as a barrier to understanding and accepting reality.

What is often overlooked in these stressful situations is that the conflict may have originated in the medical environment itself. Seriously ill patients and their loved ones receive powerful social cues from healthcare professionals and healthcare institutions, cues that suggest that the right way to behave when someone is ill is to be hopeful, and that, in particular, it is right and reasonable to place one's hopes in medical progress. It is certainly not only religious patients and loved ones who pick up on these cues; nonreligious patients may also use the language of "miracles" to capture the extraordinary, wonder-working powers of contemporary medicine. However, when a patient's condition is deteriorating, and this patient or this patient's loved ones speak of miracles, prayer, or faith—as they may have been doing all along, as individuals accustomed to framing their experience in religious or spiritual terms—healthcare professionals tend to identify the communication or decision-making problem they must now sort out as a religious problem, involving belief in divine intervention.

Professionals may be uncertain of how to respond when a surrogate or other loved one says, "*We* still have hope" during a discussion of options that include withdrawing or forgoing treatment, or when a patient asks, "Is there any hope left for me?" In such situations, to respond by asking, "Can you tell me what you hope for now?" can be helpful. It is a way for professionals to acknowledge that the language of hope and the act of hoping are familiar and important to some patients and their loved ones. It also clarifies what is being hoped for at this point. The professional who is presenting treatment options, or responding to a question about prognosis, should be prepared to explain whether a hoped-for goal is or is not attainable.

The professional should also recognize that the language of hope, and having an object for one's hopes, will continue to be important to some patients and their loved ones even when it is clear that certain once-reasonable hopes cannot be attained. Because the language of hope can be religious language or associated with religious belief and practices, the involvement of a professional chaplain can be helpful in facilitating communication during treatment decision-making and in supporting the patient and loved ones.

Sometimes different professionals involved in care of the same patient, and working from the same medical facts, will use the language of hope in conflicting or confusing ways so that a patient (or surrogate) misunderstands the patient's prognosis. This can happen even though each involved professional believes that all team members are communicating in a consistent way. Making a practice of holding medical conferences prior to family conferences can help to identify potentially confusing differences in professional vocabularies and can also help to clarify whether a patient or surrogate has, in fact, discussed hopes related to end-of-life concerns with some team members while expressing hopes for medical improvement with others.

Communications concerning hope can be further complicated by the presence of outside professionals, such as patients' own pastors, other visiting clergy, and personal physicians, whose opinion carries some authority with the patient or loved ones but who may have incomplete knowledge of the patient's prognosis and current condition, and whose goals may explicitly include encouraging hope. For this reason, ethics education concerning hope in end-of-life care settings should aim to include all categories of professionals and volunteers who may be involved in the spiritual care of community members near the end of life (Jacobs, 2010).

"LET GOD DECIDE": AMBIVALENCE, TREATMENT DECISIONS, AND RELIGIOUS LANGUAGE AND VALUES

Ambivalence on the part of a patient or surrogate concerning a decision about life-sustaining treatment is sometimes communicated through religious language—"it's all in God's hands," "let God decide." A study of professionals in intensive-care settings found that some professionals use this language themselves to signify that further efforts to intervene in the course of a disease are unlikely to benefit the patient, and that, in particular, it would be appropriate to withdraw or withhold life-sustaining technologies (Kaufman, 2005). However, professionals may not be certain whether a patient or surrogate is using this language in this way. Could a patient or surrogate be expressing a desire to continue treatment? Could a patient or surrogate be expressing a hope that someone other than the patient or surrogate will take responsibility for a decision? Does this language not express anything about the content of a decision, but rather the desire to delay making a decision, and if so, would a delay be harmful to the patient or not?

The involvement of a chaplain can be helpful if the use of religious language is a feature of a patient's or surrogate's ambivalence. Ethics consultation or conflict resolution may be required if a decision concerning treatment must be made to prevent suffering or other harm to the patient, or if clinicians need assistance in working with a surrogate when it is possible to postpone, but not indefinitely delay, a decision.

"IT'S AGAINST OUR RELIGION": RELIGIOUS OBJECTIONS DURING TREATMENT DECISION-MAKING

Some patients and surrogates will refuse medical treatments on explicitly religious objections, with the refusal of blood transfusion by patients who self-identify as Jehovah's Witnesses being the best-known example. Religious or spiritual considerations may arise in response to a proposed treatment intervention in nonspecific ways, without reference to religious doctrine but with the use of religious language. Typically, a surrogate or another loved one—sometimes a loved one who has not been closely involved in the patient's care—will object to a recommendation to forgo life-sustaining treatment by stating that to do so is "against our religion."

An objection phrased in this way may mean that a surrogate, on their own or with other loved ones, feels things are moving too fast. Some loved ones may hope that a religious objection will slow things down and buy time for further discussion. Occasionally, a loved one may assert a religious objection in order to challenge the decision-making authority of a patient or a surrogate. Some surrogates and loved ones may be particularly distressed by decisions involving artificial nutrition and hydration (ANH). A recommendation to forgo ANH on the grounds that a patient who is near death cannot benefit from and may be harmed by this technology, may feel morally wrong to the patient's loved ones and give rise to a religious objection.

In the face of such concerns or objections, more information about the nature of the objection should be obtained. A religious objection, on its own, does not constitute an informed and actionable decision. Understanding the reason or reasons for the objection, and working with the surrogate and other loved ones to clarify the goals of care as they reflect the patient's prognosis and what is known of the patient's preferences, is part of the decision-making process.

If the prospect of death will undermine a patient's or family's religious faith, any decision that acknowledges that the end of life may be near may seem morally wrong in the context of that faith tradition. This sense of death's moral wrongness is not limited to persons of religious faith, but they may be more likely to express an objection in religious terms. For a religious person, not only the loss of a loved one, but also the integrity of their own faith may seem to be at stake in a decision to forgo treatment. A person of religious faith may raise a religious objection out of a belief that continuing, not forgoing, treatment is morally wrong. Some major religions view the end of one person's bodily life as part of a continuous cycle of life, death, and rebirth, and suggest that it is wrong to use technology to confine a person in a body that is dying (Gupta & Mukherjee, 2010). In multi-faith, multi-cultural, healthcare settings, healthcare professionals should be prepared for both possibilities.

Sometimes, a relevant religious objection erupts into controversy because it was not picked up earlier in the patient's care. The routine use of a spiritual assessment tool or other standard set of questions when patients are admitted or when advance care planning is being conducted, can help prevent this problem. Research suggests that when a patient is likely to be near the end of life, regularly asking this patient and the loved ones involved in the patient's care if they are "at peace" can elicit information on sources of distress that should be remedied, and, that if undetected, can trigger conflict (Steinhauser, et al., 2006).

Inviting a surrogate and other loved ones to talk about a religious objection is not the same as asking them to quote doctrine. There may be no formal doctrine underpinning a deeply-held belief, and it may not always be possible to determine if a patient who lacks capacity shared these beliefs. Involving a chaplain as soon as a religious objection is expressed is more productive than paging the chaplain to intervene in a standoff. If the objection reflects a religious struggle or an unmet religious need among the patient's loved ones, the chaplain can collaborate with other healthcare professionals to provide support while protecting the patient's best interests and, if necessary, to provide guidance to the surrogate concerning the responsibilities of this role. If the religious objection was an effort to halt a decision-making process for some reason, the chaplain may be able to elicit the underlying source of distress and reestablish trust. Ethics consultation, conflict resolution, or both may be necessary in some cases.

Occasionally, a patient's loved ones may benefit from the involvement of their own pastor to help them sort through the religious dimensions of their objection. A collaboration between a chaplain who may be less well known to a family but more familiar with a patient's medical condition and prognosis, and a pastor who may be well known to this family but less familiar with the patient's condition and prognosis, may be helpful in such cases.

CONCLUSION

The intent of this chapter has been to support ethics education and ethical reflection in different types of healthcare institutions, including various in-patient, end-of-life care settings and hospice programs. Professionals responsible for ethics education should seek to offer educational and discussion opportunities across all professions and disciplines involved in end-of-life care, so that these opportunities are not limited to those who already self-identify with spiritual care, end-of-life care, or ethics. The issues discussed in this chapter will be most familiar to chaplains and other palliative care specialists, and perhaps to members of clinical ethics consultation teams. Clinicians who specialize in the treatment of life-threatening conditions may be less familiar with these issues and with their responsibilities and options for addressing ethical dilemmas.

In American law and custom, invoking religion tends to stop conversation or signal crisis. In end-of-life care, we must resist this tendency if we are serious about taking patients' spiritual lives seriously. We must also resist the temptation to reduce the inner life of a seriously ill person to a formula ("process," "journey," "growth," and so on), and to assume that religious faith is always a comfort, or that a dying person's spiritual care needs can be reduced to whatever spiritual care services a healthcare institution has chosen to invest in.

We must also try to overcome the fear that addressing an ethical dilemma in which religious language or religious beliefs feature is professionally risky, in that it may trigger a complaint or even legal action. Failing to address an ethical dilemma is riskier.

Nancy Berlinger, PhD, MDiv, is deputy director and research scholar at the Hastings Center, a bioethics research institute in Garrison, New York. Her research interests include end-of-life care; palliative care; ethics and policy in chronic cancer; ethics in healthcare chaplaincy; and patient safety and quality improvement. Dr. Berlinger is the author of After Harm: Medical Error and the Ethics of Forgiveness, *and project director of the forthcoming revision of the Hastings Center guidelines on end-of-life care. She is an instructor in healthcare ethics at Yale School of Nursing.*

Bruce Jennings is director of the Center for Humans and Nature, a private foundation that supports work on environmental and public health policy and planning. He is also senior consultant to the Hastings Center and teaches at the Yale School of Public Health. He has written or edited 20 books and has published more than 150 articles on bioethics and public policy issues. He is currently working on new ethical guidelines on end-of-life care under development at the Hastings Center.

REFERENCES

Balboni, T. A., Paulk, M. E., Balboni M. J., Phelps, A. C., Loggers, E. T., Wright, A. A.,...Prigerson, H. G. (2010). Provision of spiritual care to patients with advanced cancer: Associations with medical care and quality of life near death. *Journal of Clinical Oncology, 28*(3), 445–452.

de Vries, R., Berlinger, N., & Cadge, W. (2008). Lost in translation: The chaplain's role in health care. *The Hastings Center Report, 38*(6), 23–27.

Geertz, C. (1973). Religion as a cultural system. In C. Geertz (Ed.), *The interpretation of cultures: Selected essays by Clifford Geertz* (pp. 81–126). New York: Basic Books.

Gupta, V. B., & Mukherjee, D. (2010). Conflicting beliefs. *The Hasting Center Report, 40*(4), 14–15.

Harrington, S. E., & Smith, T. J. (2008). The role of chemotherapy at the end of life: When is enough, enough? *Journal of the American Medical Association, 299*(22), 2667–2678.

Jacobs, M. (2010). *Clergy guide to end-of-life issues.* Cleveland, OH: The Pilgrim Press.

Kaufman, S. (2005). *And a time to die: How American hospitals shape the end of life.* New York: Scribner.

Kleinman, A. (1988). *The illness narratives: Suffering, healing and the human condition.* NY: Basic Books.

National Hospice and Palliative Care Organization. (2001). *Guidelines for spiritual care in hospice.* Alexandria, VA: National Hospice and Palliative Care Organization.

Phelps, A. C., Maciejewski, P. K., Nilsson, M., Balboni, T. A., Wright, A. A., Paulk, M. E.,…Prigerson, H. G. (2009). Religious coping and use of intensive life-prolonging care near death in patients with advanced cancer. *Journal of the American Medical Association, 301*(11), 1140–1147.

Quill, T. E., Arnold, R. M., & Platt, F. (2001). "I wish things were different": Expressing wishes in response to loss, futility, and unrealistic hopes. *Annals of Internal Medicine, 135*(7), 551–555.

Robinson, M., Thiel, M., Backus, M., & Meyer E. (2006). Matters of spirituality at the end of life in the pediatric intensive care unit. *Pediatrics, 118*(3), 719–729.

Smith, T. J., Dow, L. A., Virago, E., Khatcheressian, J., Lyckholm, L. J., & Matsuyama, R. (2010). Giving honest information to patients with advanced cancer maintains hope. *Oncology, 24*(6), 521–525.

Steinhauser, K. E., Voils, C. I., Clipp, E. C., Bosworth, H. B., Christakis, N. A., & Tulsky, J. A. (2006). "Are you at peace?": One item to probe spiritual concerns at the end of life. *Archives of Internal Medicine, 166,* 101–105.

CHAPTER 5

The Role of Ritual at the End of Life

Pamela Baird

R ituals are an integral part of human life. People the world over, regardless of age, culture, gender, socioeconomic status, religious affiliation, or spiritual beliefs engage in rituals every day. Rituals are so common they are often not identified as rituals at all, but merely called familiar everyday occurrences: the morning cup of coffee, the nightly bedtime story, the family picnic every 4th of July, or saying grace before dinner. Rituals are not only fundamental to the ordinary moments of daily living, but are extremely important and beneficial in times of tragedy, illness, and death (Anderson, 2003).

DEFINITIONS AND DESCRIPTIONS OF RITUAL

So what is a ritual? The *American Heritage Dictionary* states that a ritual is "the body of ceremonies or rites used in a place of worship" (2010). Like this definition, the most common use of the word pertains to religious beliefs and doctrine. These rituals, many instituted hundreds or even thousands of years ago, are well-known, well-loved traditions that provide solace, strength, and comfort to many.

In the same source, ritual is also defined as "a ceremonial act or a series of such acts" (2010). This kind of ritual is not always generated out of years of tradition but is often original and spontaneously created. These kinds of ceremonies or rituals can be created by patients or loved ones searching to make sense of the world, struggling to find meaning, and exploring ways to come to grips with a terminal diagnosis or impending death. These unique, individualized ceremonial acts are also common in the grief process among family members and friends who are mourning the death of a loved one.

According to anthropologist Angeles Arrien, "Ritual is recognizing a life change, and doing something to honor and support the change" (1993, p. 113). Thomas Moore wrote in *The Education of the Heart* that "any action that speaks to the soul and to the deep imagination, whether or not it also has practical effects, is a ritual...even the smallest rites of everyday existence are important to the soul" (1997, p. 111).

Theologian Megory Anderson, an authority on creating personalized rituals for the dying, says:

> When I vigil with the dying, I sometimes use formal religious rites from specific faith traditions—the last rites—but more often I create rituals of my own, drawing from the circumstances of each situation. Rituals are meant to be ageless and timeless, bringing the needs of the participants into the present situation. (2003, p. *xx*)

All of these definitions and expressions are cogent to this discussion of the role of ritual at the end of life. There are timeless rituals: sitting shiva, offering prescribed prayers, the anointing of the sick, chanting mantras, meditation, or reciting of the Psalms. And there are newly created personalized rituals, crafted to support and serve those who are in need at the present moment. Whether these rituals have endured through the millennia or have recently been brought to life, their value is measured in how much healing, connection, and meaning they deliver to the participants.

DEFINITIONS: RELIGIOUS AND SPIRITUAL

In this chapter the terms *spiritual* and *religious* will be used. These terms have often been used interchangeably, implying that they are the same. However, the literature is moving in the direction of defining them separately. To date, there has been no agreed upon definition of *spiritual* or *spirituality* (Baird, 2010). For the purpose of this chapter, the definition used is the one crafted by a consensus conference in February 2009. This group came together "to establish a common language and model for interdisciplinary spiritual care..." (Puchalski & Ferrell, 2010, p. *xxi*). Forty national leaders were invited, including "physicians, nurses, psychologists, social workers, chaplains and clergy, other spiritual care providers, and healthcare administrators" (p. *xxi*). The definition they wrote and agreed upon was:

> Spirituality is the aspect of humanity that refers to the way individuals seek and express meaning and purpose, and the way they experience their connectedness to the moment, to self, to others, to nature and to the significant or sacred. (p. 25)

For the purpose of this chapter, *religious* is defined as "pertaining to an organization that has a set of rites, rules, practices, values, and beliefs that prescribe how individuals should live their lives and respond to God" (Thoresen, 1999).

Spirituality and religiosity are very personal. Many families have strictly followed a specific religious teaching for generations. Many individuals in those families would never consider any other way of expressing their spirituality and proudly consider themselves faithfully religious. Still others in those same families choose not to follow the family's traditional ways and would not identify themselves as religious. And there are families who have never believed in, or practiced, any religious teaching and would certainly not use the term religious to describe themselves. Using the stated definition of spirituality, everyone is considered spiritual because all people seek and express meaning and purpose, and experience connectedness to the moment, to self, to others, to nature, and to the significant or sacred.

WHAT RITUALS PROVIDE AND WHY WE USE THEM

Rituals provide connection. They connect us to the moment, to ourselves, to others, to nature, and to the significant or sacred. Rituals at their core are spiritual in nature. Rituals, these spiritual expressions, are created from the human need for connection. Religions across the world have recognized this need and have utilized ritual since religion began. Much like life preservers, rituals can be something to hang on to when the world feels unrecognizable and seems to be falling apart. In times of joy and celebration and in uncertainty and fear, rituals can be a source of connection.

Rituals also help us make sense of the world and can be a link to finding meaning in what sometimes feels like a meaningless sea of pain and suffering. A diagnosis of cancer, ALS, dementia, or any catastrophic illness can turn life upside down and create uncertainty of the future and fear of the unknown. People often respond to a terminal diagnosis with the question "Why?" Human beings want to know the "why" of things and search endlessly for meaning in common everyday events, happy occasions, or times of trouble. Rituals are "a practical way of dealing with some specific circumstances" (Bell, 2009, p. 92).

Rituals also provide healing. Perhaps one the most frequently used rituals is prayer. From many wide-ranging belief systems, people pray in search of physical, social, psychological, and spiritual healing. It is important to clarify that *healing* and *cure* are not synonymous. Jeanne Achterberg says of healing:

1. Healing is a lifelong journey toward wholeness.
2. Healing is remembering what has been forgotten about connection, and unity and interdependence among all things living and nonliving.
3. Healing is embracing what is most feared.
4. Healing is opening what has been closed, softening what has hardened into obstruction.
5. Healing is entering into the transcendent, timeless moment when one experiences the divine.
6. Healing is creativity and passion and love.
7. Healing is seeking and expressing self in its fullness, its light and shadow, its male and female.
8. Healing is learning to trust life. (Achterberg, 1990, p. 194)

ELEMENTS OF EFFECTIVE RITUALS

There is no set formula for rituals. Rituals and ceremonial acts vary greatly and can be: deliberate and planned; free flowing and organic; structured with a beginning, middle, and end; spontaneous and impromptu; repetitious and designed to be done over and over; or experienced only once.

There is very little agreement upon "the intrinsic features of ritual" (Bell, 2009, p. 91), although there are some elements that seem to be universal. Some of the elements most commonly used are: candles, dance, feathers, food, herbs, incense, music, oil, prayer, rocks or shells, silence, song, storytelling, and water.

Long practiced religious traditions have very prescribed ways to use elements in rituals and often these elements are as important as the ritual itself. Personal rituals afford the creator the opportunity to choose what elements, if any, are used, and how best to use them. Whether the elements used in the ritual have their roots in religion or are chosen spontaneously in the moment, their purpose is to help us make sense of the world, find connection and meaning, and experience healing.

RITUALS IN ANTICIPATION OF DEATH

The need for ritual can be strong when facing the end of life. Everyone responds to death in different ways. For some, anticipation of death creates feelings of devastation and hopelessness. For others, it can bring about transformation. Whether the result is devastation, transformation, or something in between, preparation for death can be supported by the use of rituals (Arrien, 1993, p. 113).

Upon hearing a terminal prognosis, some people find refuge in things that are familiar. Connecting or reconnecting with the religious faith and teachings of childhood or engaging in familiar traditions and rituals can sometimes bring relief to a shattered world. Sitting in familiar pews, praying toward Mecca five times a day, praying with sacred beads, reading holy texts, chanting familiar words—these and numerous other religious rituals are life-affirming and can mean the difference between feeling helpless or resilient. Some who turn to well-used religious rituals find they are calmed by the familiarity and repetition of age-old traditions (Anderson, 2003, p. 25).

As stated before, for those who are nonreligious, the familiarity and repetition of traditional religious rituals may not provide a sense of connection, meaning, or healing. Sometimes part of the benefit of the ritual is the ability to create something new and unique—something meaningful in this particular moment, under these specific circumstances.

The 2007 film *The Bucket List* told the story of two men with cancer who created a list of things they wanted to do before they died. A lot of people, even before the movie was released, have felt the same need to create a "bucket list": things to do before you "kick the bucket." These lists vary as much as the individuals who write them. Some make plans to climb a magnificent mountain or parachute from an airplane while others dream of sitting at the beach with family and friends enjoying every last sunset.

Every day somewhere, a grandmother calls together her family to ritualistically pass on her favorite possessions to her children and grandchildren. One grandfather who was imminently dying gathered his family for one last visit. The adult children shared stories and memories with their father. The grandchildren sang, danced, and recited poems for him. The 2-day celebration of his life was filled with Grandpa's favorite foods, culminating with hot fudge sundaes—a family favorite—in the wee hours of the morning.

One family spent a few days with video cameras, interviewing the elderly grandparents and documenting their lives, hopes, and dreams. Less than 2 months after they completed the project, the grandfather began showing definite signs of dementia, which shows that sooner is often better than later when planning rituals at the end of life.

Inspired by *The Four Things That Matter Most*, some facing the end of life have contacted specific people to say, "Please forgive me," "I forgive you," "Thank you," and "I love you" (Byock, 2004).

Some rituals aren't planned ahead of time but are created in the moment. Sometimes the time just feels right and the one who is dying is in the mood to talk and reminisce. Sharing stories, life review, and looking through photo albums are rituals that serve to create connections to family and friends and memories of the past.

Even when people are hospitalized, rituals of all kinds can be used—planned or spontaneous. A chaplain was on her way out the door one evening when she was paged to the room of a 35-year-old woman a few days from death. The woman's parents were at her bedside and had called the chaplain to ask for prayer. The patient, it turned out, was not particularly interested in praying, but did want something from the chaplain. A few weeks before, this young woman had lost the ability to talk. Nevertheless, it was the week before Christmas and what she wanted at that moment was to sing Christmas carols. Unable to speak, she found a way to squeak out sounds enough so that her mother and the chaplain understood which songs she wanted to sing. And so, for the better part of the evening, the three women sang song after song, accompanied at times by nurses, phlebotomists, and other hospital workers who came in to give care and to join in the singing. One needed only to see the smile on her face that night to recognize the power of the ritual of song. That was the last time the young woman ever sang (Baird, 2010, p. 668).

Rituals Near the Time of Death

There are a number of rituals, both religious and nonreligious, that are commonly used at the time of death. Here again, because death can be so unnerving, people often gravitate to the familiar. Fondly remembered childhood experiences can provide a sense of relief and peace even if religion hasn't been a part of their lives for many years. It is very common for patients to involve religious practitioners and chaplains as death draws near. Frequently, patients and families seek the comfort of religious rituals: the anointing of the sick, chanting, communion, confession, meditation, prayers, reciting mantras, singing, and any number of other religious practices (Fosarelli, 2008).

Not all rituals performed at the bedsides of the dying are religious in nature. Many are spontaneous, relative to the situation. Perhaps one of the most universal rituals at the time of death is the coming together of family and friends. It is not uncommon to see a number of people gather, each taking turns sitting with the dying and then going outside the sickroom to support one another.

This common, everyday ritual serves many purposes. It can be a time for both the dying and their family members to speak any last words. For some people there are things they have been longing to say for years and only at this moment do they find the courage to speak the words. This bedside ritual can also provide the occasion to look into the other's eyes and to say goodbye. It can also be beneficial for family members and friends as they meet, reconnect, and support one another.

A 45-year-old woman was dying in a cancer hospital where she had been a patient for several years. She was a longtime member of a Christian church and had been supported by the people in her church through the cancer treatment. When word reached the parishioners she was dying, 20 people stood around her bed one evening and sweetly sang to her for the better part of the evening.

RITUALS IMMEDIATELY AFTER DEATH

Just after death, it is not uncommon for family and friends to, once again, gather to say their last goodbyes. Some people pray, some bring flowers, others laugh and tell stories, and still others stand silent. For the religious, there can be many rules or religious laws that need to be followed. Many religions have a set of specific guidelines for the time of death. How strictly the religious rituals are followed is usually determined by how observant the person was or how important the rituals are to the family members.

Some traditions require the body be left in place for a period of minutes, hours, or even days. Some require burial; others prefer cremation. Some teachings say the body must be buried within 24 hours. Others feel the need to wait at least 3 days before the body is cremated.

A hundred years ago, when almost everyone died at home, preparing the body was left to the family, friends, and religious community. Today, with most people dying in hospitals or nursing homes, this task is generally done by nursing assistants who may never have even met the one who died and may not be aware of any significant rituals. This is important because some religions have specific rules about who can wash the body: anyone; anyone of the same gender; anyone of the same faith; or only a male of the same faith. Washing the body is only one of many rituals at the time of death but it certainly seems to be an important one. Given how much is written about washing and preparing the body, it is apparent that many feel this ritual to be a sacred act.

Knowing how important it is to properly care for the body and how difficult it can be for parents of children who die, one children's hospital chaplain created a ritual for parents who want to wash and hold their child's body one last time. The chaplain is prepared to assist in the ritual at the parents' request. A special box is made for each family. Each box, beautifully and lovingly assembled, contains washcloths, a soft blanket, anointing oil, a little cloth bag to hold a piece of the child's hair, and written prayers. Music is available if the family chooses. The parents are encouraged to follow their own instincts and their hearts as they wash their child's body—and to take as much time as they need. Every effort is made to support the parents and follow their lead in this ritual as they say goodbye to their child.

The days and weeks after death are filled with rituals as well. Funerals, memorial services, burial, cremation, placing headstones, receiving visits, letters, phone calls, and food from friends are all familiar rituals.

RITUALS IN BEREAVEMENT

There are many rituals that support people in their grief. Some religions are very specific and define the mourning period, specific times during the year to honor the dead, what clothes and activities are appropriate, and what prayers and readings should be recited for those who mourn. For both the religious and nonreligious who want to create rituals specific to this moment in life, there are countless ways to ritualize grief.

A few weeks after the memorial service, one family, seven in number, traveled 400 miles to a place on the California coast that was loved by their wife and mother who died. She had been cremated and wanted her ashes scattered along the seaside and in the ocean. Her husband divided her ashes into seven small pouches. When the family arrived at their destination, it was raining and they ate their picnic lunch in the car. Just as they finished, the rain stopped, the skies began to clear, and a rainbow framed the horizon. Each one took a pouch and walked alone to distant parts of the beach, said their own private goodbyes and released the ashes of their wife and mother onto seaside and into the sea. This ritual provided unanticipated healing to this family whose loved one had died unexpectedly and without warning.

Some rituals might require driving 400 miles, but most do not. Healing and connection can be found in simple ways: listening to the favorite music of the one who died; planting a tree or a garden in memory; sitting in the loved one's favorite chair; doing something helpful or honorable in the person's memory.

Near the conclusion of memorial services, a minister often asks the family and friends to bring to mind that one quality they admired most in the one who died. He or she then invites them to begin, this very day, to incorporate that quality into their own lives, adding that it is a way to show their love, keep the departed close to their hearts, and to make the world a better place.

While every religion and tradition is unique in the way grief is ritualized, there are some commonalities: to respect and support those who are grieving; to stay in contact with the bereaved; and food. Food may seem an unusual choice here but food brings people together—and food is love. Throughout the ages, societies have created numerous rituals around food. Perhaps one of the most common is taking food to the bereaved. Food is a necessity of life and a simple demonstration of concern and caring. As with all rituals, the importance and the power lies in the connection, meaning, and healing it provides.

CONCLUSION

> There are aspects of grieving that are personal and aspects that are shared. There are aspects of grieving that live in our hearts and minds and have no need of expression. And there are aspects of grieving that call for, yearn for, expression. That is the moment we turn to ritual. (Coryell, 1998, p. 109)

The end of life, in its mystery and uncertainty, can cause us to lose our way for a time. Rituals have a powerful way of helping us regain our balance. For as long as anyone can remember, rituals, both religious and spontaneous, have been vital to our humanity. We are spiritual beings who in this human experience long for connectedness, making sense of things, finding meaning, and healing. Rituals make it possible.

Rev. Pamela Baird is an ordained minister who serves as an end-of-life practitioner providing end-of-life training to both medical professionals and laypersons in the community. After working for many years as a hospice and hospital chaplain, in 2008, Rev. Baird created Seasons of Life, an innovative community-based program to explore the nature of suffering and the spiritual and existential issues experienced at the end of life. She also serves as a consultant on research projects with the Nursing Research & Education Division at City of Hope. Rev. Baird has authored writings on spirituality and palliative care. She is a graduate of the Metta Institute End-of-Life Practitioner Program and is a recipient of the Southern California Cancer Pain Initiative (SCCPI) Award of Excellence in Pain Management.

REFERENCES

Achterberg, J. (1990). *Woman as healer.* Boston, MA: Shambhala Publications.

Anderson, M. (2003). *Sacred dying.* New York: Marlowe & Company.

Arrien, A. (1993). *The four-fold way.* New York: Harper Collins.

Baird, P. (2010). Spiritual care interventions. In B. R. Ferrell & N. Coyle (Eds.), *Oxford textbook of palliative nursing* (pp. 663–671). New York: Oxford University Press.

Bell, C. (2009). *Ritual theory, ritual practice.* New York: Oxford University Press.

Byock, I. (2004). *The four things that matter most.* New York: Free Press.

Coryell, D. M. (1998). *Good grief.* Santa Fe, NM: The Shiva Foundation.

Fosarelli, P. (2008). *Prayers & rituals at a time of illness & dying.* West Conshohocken, PA: Templeton Foundation Press.

Moore, T. (1997). *The education of the heart.* New York: Harper Perennial.

Puchalaski, C. M., & Ferrell, B. R. (2010). *Making health care whole.* West Conshohocken, PA: Templeton Press.

The American Heritage Dictionary of the English Language. (2010). Retrieved from http://education.yahoo.com/reference/dictionary/entry/ritual

Thoresen, E. C. (1999). Spirituality and health: Is there a relationship? *Health Psychology, 4*(3), 409–431.

CHAPTER 6

Legacy and Spirituality at the End Of Life

Gary S. Fink

Spirituality is often conceived as mysterious and other-worldly, but it is not necessarily so. Spirituality can be divined through day-to-day existence—in who we are, in what we do, and in the totality of our lives—in other words, through legacy. We confront our finitude at the end of life, contemplating the life we have lived, relationships with people and the world around us, and the meaning of our existence. These spiritual issues may evoke anxiety, uncertainty, or distress. Legacy work provides a powerful and important tool for practitioners to address existential and spiritual concerns in the face of terminal illness and impending death (Hunter, 2007–2008).

Legacy is an aspect of the self that remains in the world after death. A legacy is sometimes something specific that we leave for others after our death (Hunter, 2007–2008; Hunter & Rowles, 2005). In the broadest sense, however, legacy refers to the sum total of the life we have lived. I will focus mainly on that broad view of legacy—that is, legacy as the impact or influence of our lives in the world.

LEGACY AND SPIRITUALITY

Legacy work involves the two essential aspects of spirituality—a sense of meaning and purpose, and transcendent connections (Puchalski et al., 2009). Legacy building affirms meaning within a person's life and the value of the life lived. Consciously or unconsciously, individuals weave their discrete memories into a meaningful tapestry, creating a personal narrative—a life story—that is built upon experiences, goals, values, and lessons learned from life (Johnson, 2003).

Legacy building also affirms connections that transcend death. Terminally ill individuals may find comfort and reassurance in the hope or anticipation that their influence or impact in the world will remain after their death. Individuals can attain a kind of immortality through gifts of words, ideas, values, or objects, and in continued bonds that loved ones feel (Lifton, 1979). Transcendent connections may also be found in an individual's identification with a particular group, such as extended family, an ethnic group, or a faith community.

MEANING-MAKING AT THE END OF LIFE

Meaning-making is an essential task of legacy building that provides a way to address fundamental spiritual questions: "How have I made a difference in the world?" "What is the value of my life?" "What is my place and purpose in the universe?" Psychologist Erik Erikson asserts that the last stage of psychosocial development deals with the existential issue of *ego integrity* versus *despair* (Erikson, 1959). "Ego integrity is defined as a basic acceptance of one's life as having been inevitable, appropriate, and meaningful" (Haber, 2006, p. 157). In order to make sense of the totality of our existence, we must decide and define what is meaningful about our lives. McAdams (1993) theorizes that "we create a self that is whole and purposeful because it is embedded in a coherent and meaningful story....We create myth so that our lives, and the lives of others, will make sense" (p. 92).

A life story—specifically, how an individual perceives the meaning of his life—can be used in both assessment and treatment of spiritual distress at the end of life. Clinical use of the life story can address a range of end-of-life crises that arise from the initial terminal diagnosis to the time of death and throughout the grieving process. "Those who work with the aging population or those faced with a life-threatening illness must be aware of the importance of passing along one's 'self,' of making meaning" (Hunter, 2007–2008, p. 327). Narrative approaches to therapy are often utilized to understand how people make sense of adversity and personally evolve (McAdams, 2006). Through the emerging life story, whether told by someone or spoken about someone, the spiritual care provider can help identify issues that need to be addressed. Spiritual issues that may cause suffering at the end of life include guilt, forgiveness, personal worth and value, meaning of affliction, relationship with a higher power, yearning for faith or hope, and unfinished business. Existential crises that arise at the end of life provide opportunities for creative interventions—particularly around legacy building—that promote empowerment and provide comfort to clients when their worlds are in disarray (Otis-Green, 2003). A narrative, life story approach to spiritual care can be a useful tool for assessment, analysis, and intervention at the end of life without evoking the social stigma sometimes associated with psychiatry and psychotherapy (Weiss, 1995; Haight et al., 2003).

IMPACT OF MEANING-MAKING

Finding or creating coherence in one's life is one of many benefits that emerge from the meaning-making process. Additionally, meaning-making activities may affirm a sense of personal value; promote self-acceptance; and enhance self-affirmation, self-esteem, and confidence (Chiang, 2008). The process of meaning-making may also facilitate coming to terms with life and death, with painful memories or experiences, and may enhance relationships with significant others.

Meaning-making activities help individuals from diverse spiritual orientations come to terms with life and death. Some individuals profess a religious faith that their lives and the universe have an order and purpose that come from God or a higher power. Other individuals may discern no transcendent meaning in life and perceive no overarching purpose to existence, yet come to view their own particular lives as meaningful. "Meaning of life" is not the same as "meaning of *my* life" (Yalom, 1980). One can be deeply committed to living a purposeful life in the universe without believing that life has a universal purpose.

Some patients draw upon a preexistent spiritual orientation or assumptive world that offers ways to make sense of suffering, find strength and comfort, and sustain hope in some form. In that case, the counselor may validate and reinforce beliefs that provide grace at the end of life. Other patients, however, may not draw any meaning or value from spiritual distress, emotional pain, or physical suffering. In those cases, exploring the meaning of suffering, anxiety, or guilt in the mind and life of a patient offers opportunities to integrate the end-of-life experience into the context of the patient's life (Breitbart, Gibson, Poppito, & Berg, 2004).

Meaning-making activities facilitate coming to terms with painful memories of past events. An array of literature associates positive outcomes with disclosure of stressful or negative emotional experiences (Steinhauser et al., 2008). Recalling negative experiences may help patients view the past with new perspectives to facilitate healing (Pennebaker & Seagal, 1999) as individuals articulate, acknowledge, evaluate, and integrate difficult past events into a larger psychosocial and spiritual context (Graybeal, Sexton, & Pennebaker, 2002). As a result, individuals are able to frame or reframe the meaning of an emotion-laden event within the larger framework of their life experience (Steinhauser et al., 2008).

Meaning-based coping (Folkman, 1997) can diminish the impact of negative life experiences through adjustment of goals and expectations, focus on positive events, and spiritual belief. Meaning-making activities may strengthen, reaffirm, or repair personal relationships. For many, the end of life is a welcome time to share appreciation, affection, and blessings with loved ones. However, when guilt, pain, or distress is associated with a significant other, individuals may wish to come to terms with negative emotions previously avoided or denied. The end of life provides an opportunity to resolve unfinished business (Otis-Green, 2003) and come to terms with emotional hardships and painful circumstances such as alcoholism, abuse, or parental aloofness (Hunter, 2007–2008). Spiritual traditions offer prescribed ways to create new meanings from old wounds. Creative spiritual rituals may also be useful in reframing negative relationships. Meaning-making activities provide opportunities to atone, forgive, reconcile, or move beyond difficult personal relationships.

CONTINUING BONDS: GENERATIVITY

Legacy work expands the way we think about afterlife. Typically, discussions of life after death include the idea of heaven as a place where souls reside. A 2005 ABC News poll indicated that most Christians in the United States envision continued existence in a heavenly, other-worldly place after death. Legacy, on the other hand, provides "this-worldly" possibilities that life can transcend death. It provides a way to ensure a continuing presence in this world and leave something meaningful behind. For those whose spiritual worldview may not envision or emphasize a supernatural afterlife, practices of legacy building may diminish existential anxiety arising from life's finitude. The hope of continuing existence through continued bonds or ongoing influence in this world may offer comfort at the end of life. Erikson hypothesizes that the next-to-last stage of personal development focuses on generativity: the need to create a positive legacy that lives on after death—to leave a part of the self to future generations to help guide their lives (Erikson, 1963). In many cultures and spiritual traditions, continued bonds with those who have died are expressed and preserved through rituals, folkways, and customs.

CONTINUING BONDS: EMOTIONAL RELOCATION

Holding on to the legacy of a loved one who has died facilitates emotional relocation of the deceased in the mind of survivors, enhancing healthy grieving. William Worden writes that an essential task of grief is to "emotionally relocate the deceased," recognizing the necessity of continuing bonds (Worden, 2002, p. 15–16). Successful grieving, then, involves a paradox—both holding on and letting go. Maintaining continuing bonds with the deceased helps a mourner to move on with life. Particularly among bereaved children, maintaining an identification with deceased parents is an important part of the bereavement process (Silverman & Nickman, 1996), along with investment in new relationships (Tyson-Rawson, 1996). The transmission of legacy helps significant others establish new forms of continuing bonds with the deceased (McClement et al., 2007), and helps maintain a transcendent and ongoing relationship with a loved one no longer alive.

RESPECTFUL REGARD

Articulating and creating legacy reinforces self-worth for a person at the end of life and enhances respectful regard for that person. Building a legacy that embodies a person's past and present underscores the value of a life lived. Finding or creating meaning in someone's life story is a profound life-affirming process that validates a person's very existence and the unique value of each individual's life (Garland & Garland, 2001). A spiritual consciousness, whether religious or secular, affirms that every life counts and that every person has inherent sacred value. Legacy building increases the patient's understanding at the end of life and enhances his or her relationships with caregivers and family members (Phillips, 2010). In institutional settings, legacy activities personalize patients and promote equity between the caregiver and the recipient of care.

REMINISCENCE THERAPY

Reminiscence in its simplest form is remembering the past. Reminiscence therapy is a treatment modality in which the counselor encourages the patient to recall and share memories and experiences from the past (Miller, 2009). Simple questions about past experiences may produce a stream of memories. Prompts such as photos (Sherman, 1995), period music (Kartman, 1991), and family trees may be useful (Butler, 1963, 1974; Doka, 1993).

Reminiscence therapy can be utilized in a variety of settings and offers many clinical options for the counselor. Reminiscence is an effective tool to strengthen the therapeutic alliance between counselor and patient (Miller, 2009). It can involve individuals, families, or groups, and can be facilitated formally or informally. Topics may include "family and friendships, loves and losses, achievements and disappointments, and adjustments to life's changes (p.8)." Reminiscence is used to address many spiritual challenges including coping with life's disappointments and fostering appreciation for life's blessings. Reminiscing fosters communication and self-esteem, and has been shown to enhance mood, particularly among patients with depression (Serrano,

Latorre, Gatz, & Montanes, 2004). Recalling personal experiences, struggles, and triumphs validates and affirms a person's life which is fundamentally threatened by impending death. Although side effects of reminiscence therapy are minimal (Miller, 2009), counselors should exercise caution, as stressful or deeply painful memories may be difficult to process effectively given the limitations imposed by a patient's condition, terminal diagnosis, or cognitive impairment.

LIFE REVIEW THERAPY

Life review therapy is a powerful way to facilitate legacy building and spiritual meaning-making for an individual facing the end of life (Butler, 1963; Johnson, 2003). Life review is a form of reminiscence (Haight et al., 2003) that goes beyond recalling of past events and experiences to include a more structured review and reframing of a person's life history (Burnside & Haight, 1992). Reminiscence is usually characterized as a descriptive process; life review is considered more evaluative. Haber (2006) notes that "participants examine how their memories contribute to the meaning of their life, and they may work at coming to terms with more difficult memories" (p.154).

In life review, the counselor assists the reviewer in assembling and organizing memories into a coherent, comprehensive narrative (Haight et al., 2003), and reconstructing the past in order to facilitate meaning-making (Worden, 2002; Wallace, 1992). It involves reframing of the past (Sadavoy & Lazarus, 2000) to more gracefully confront and more effectively cope with the end of life. Life stories often revolve around themes, such as struggles of ancestors, identity, turning points, new beginnings, challenges, and achievements (Hunter, 2007–2008; Haber, 2006).

The positive effect of forgiveness on spiritual well-being is an increasingly popular area of research (Steinhauser et al., 2008; Lawler et al., 2005). Some spiritual perspectives view forgiveness as an act of grace granted by the victim to the offender. Other spiritual orientations view forgiveness not as something given, but as something found—a state of being that is achieved. Forgiveness becomes a process of letting go of past resentments rather than absolving another person's bad behavior (Byock, 2004). The focus is not on recounting rights and wrongs, but on mitigating emotional consequences of feeling wronged.

Life review can be done by a variety of people in a number of ways. Activity directors, students, as well as volunteers initiate life review opportunities under the supervision of instructors and volunteer managers (Haber, 2006).

Life reviews may be conducted orally with recording devices, though written versions increase efficacy and positive impact (Sherman, 1991, 1995). Concluding the life review process with a tangible product, such as a memory book, written biography or autobiography, or video increases its positive effect (Johnson, 2003; Haight et al. 2003).

Life review therapy has been shown to lessen symptoms of spiritual and emotional suffering, particularly at the end of life. Beneficial effects include reduction of depression and anxiety (Bohlmeijer, Smit, & Cuijpers, 2003; Erlin, Mellors, Sereika, & Cook, 2001; Haight, Michel, & Hendrix, 1998), as well as greater spiritual well-being (Ando, Morita, Okamoto, & Ninosaka, 2008). Therapeutic life review can bolster the ability to cope with loss, guilt, conflict, or defeat, and can help individuals find meaning in life accomplishments (Haber, 2006). Individuals find greater self-regard, sense of purpose, and quality of life through life review activities (Haight, Michel, & Hendrix, 1998; Erlin, Mellors, Sereika, & Cook 2001).

The impact of life review is not confined to the person confronting death. Because it can be used to promote generativity and continuing bonds in a variety of ways, family members and others benefit from the tangible and intangible gifts that emerge from the life review process long after the patient's death.

The following resources may be helpful in preparing a life review:

- Birren, J. E., & Birren, B. A. (1996). Autobiography: Exploring the self and encouraging development. In J. E. Birren, G. M. Kenyon, J. E. Ruth, J. J. F. Schroots, & T. Svensson (Eds.), *Aging and biography: Explorations in adult development* (283–299). New York: Springer.
- Haight, B. K., & Webster, J. D. (Eds.). (1995). *The art and science of reminiscing: Theory, research methods, and applications.* Bristol, PA: Taylor & Francis.
- Hospice Foundation of America. (1999). *A guide to recalling and telling your life story.* Washington, DC: Hospice Foundation of America.
- Hospice Memory Book Program. (1998). Weaverville, CA: Boulden.

DIGNITY THERAPY

Dignity therapy (Chochinov et al., 2005) is a meaning-making intervention directed toward patients and families involving life-affirmation and legacy-building. After 6–8 sessions of recalling and discussing life experiences guided by a clinician, a *generativity document* is written and produced. Dignity enhancement therapy addresses a number of spiritual and psychological issues, including autonomy and control, self-esteem, continuity of the self in the face of mortality, role preservation, maintenance of hope, legacy, and generativity (Chochinov et al., 2005; Steinhauser et al., 2008).

During therapy sessions, patients discuss issues that are most salient to them and are encouraged to identify what they hope will be remembered after their death. These conversations are recorded, transcribed, edited, and finally presented to family members or loved ones. The goals of creating this generativity document are to reduce suffering and enhance a patient's sense of purpose, meaning, dignity, and quality of life (McClement et al., 2007). In addition, the generativity document is intended to ease distress and provide comfort during the grief process for those who are bereaved.

McClement and colleagues (2007) write that dignity therapy "provides a potential enduring bridge between the patient and surviving family, offering solace and support at the end stages of the patient's life and during the bereavement period." (p. 1080) Patients nearing death report greater sense of meaning, hope, purpose, and dignity (Chochinov et al., 2005). Family members report that dignity therapy eases suffering and distress associated with bereavement. Survivors find comfort in affirming the life of their loved one (McClement et al., 2007), and are better able to transform their attachment into continuing bonds of memory and legacy (Boerner & Heckhausen, 2003).

ETHICAL WILLS

In recent years, the practice of writing an ethical will has become a popular and useful tool to create a legacy that provides reassurance of continued presence and influence after death while providing family members and significant others with continued bonds to a deceased loved one. Ethical wills are documents or testimonies prepared before death that contain reflections, blessings, instructions, personal histories, or values to be passed on to others.

Ethical wills originate in Biblical literature as family blessings. In medieval times, writers added personal histories, important values, and ethical beliefs. For European Jews, ethical wills became a means of transmitting precious moral legacies, especially at times of persecution in which material assets were threatened. Usually, ethical wills were written in the format of letters to loved ones—providing opportunities to communicate with loved ones after death.

Otis-Green (2003) encourages counselors and therapists to embrace the legacy interests of those at the end of life by offering guidance in preparation of ethical wills. Individuals near the end of life or confronted by terminal illness can create letters, videotapes, or audio recordings to pass on to significant others (Johnson, 2003). Ethical wills can be simple—though not always easy—to prepare with or without the guidance of a trained counselor and can be customized to reflect cultural norms and personal styles and abilities.

The following resources may be helpful to guide preparation of ethical wills:

- Baines, B. (2001). *Ethical wills: Putting your values on paper*. Cambridge, MA: Perseus.
- Greiff, B. S. (1999). *Legacy: The giving of life's greatest treasures: Loving, learning, laboring, laughing, lamenting, linking, living, leading, and leaving*. New York: Harper Collins/Regan Books.
- McPhelimy, L. (1997). *In the checklist of life: A "working book" to help you live and leave this life* (2nd ed.). Rockfall, CT: AAIP Publishing.
- Riemer, J., & Stampfer, N. (1991). *So that your values live on: Ethical wills and how to prepare them*. Woodstock, VT: Jewish Lights.
- Sheridan, J. (2009). The ethical will: A modern approach to an ancient tradition. *LLI Review, 4*, 114–120.

Conclusion

Legacy work promotes spiritual well-being for patients and their loved ones, particularly at the end of life. Legacy building fosters transcendent meaning and connections in life and in death. It focuses on meaningful aspects of the self that will remain in the world after death and reflects three life-affirming principles: that every life counts, that it is never too late for repentance or reconciliation, and that every life makes a difference.

Rabbi Gary S. Fink, D.Min., is a pastoral counselor who specializes in bereavement, loss, and life-limiting illness. He serves as chaplain at Montgomery Hospice in Rockville, Maryland, and as project coordinator for the Montgomery Hospice Dementia Initiative, providing education and training for professional caregivers and families of people with dementia. Rabbi Fink teaches in the Psychology Graduate Program at Hood College in Frederick, Maryland, and conducts classes in Ethics for the Florence Melton Continuing Education program. He was named Rabbi Emeritus of Oseh Shalom Congregation in recognition of more than 25 years of service in the congregational ministry. Rabbi Fink was ordained at Hebrew Union College and earned a Doctorate of Ministry at the Howard University School of Divinity, concentrating in end-of-life care and counseling. He holds a graduate Certificate in Thanatology.

REFERENCES

ABC News Poll, December 20, 2005. Retrieved July 10, 2010 from http://abcnews.go.com/images/Politics/994a1Heaven.pdf

Allen, R. S., Hilgeman, M. M., Ege, M. A., Shuster, J. L., & Burgio, L. D. (2008). Legacy activities as interventions approaching the end of life. *Journal of Palliative Medicine, 11*(7), 1029–1038.

Ando, M., Morita, T., Okamoto, T., & Ninosaka, Y. (2008). One-week short-term life review interview can improve spiritual well-being of terminally ill cancer patients. *Psycho-Oncology, 17,* 885–890.

Baines, B. (2001). *Ethical wills: Putting your values on paper.* Cambridge, MA: Perseus.

Bauer, J. J., McAdams, D. P., & Pals, J. L. (2008). Narrative identity and eudaimonic well-being. *Journal of Happiness Studies, 9,* 81–104.

Boerner, K., & Heckhausen, J. (2003). To have and have not: Adaptive bereavement by transforming mental ties to the deceased. *Death Studies, 27,* 199–226.

Bohlmeijer, E., Smit, F., & Cuijpers, P. (2003). Effects of reminiscence and life review on late life depression: A meta-analysis. *International Journal of Geriatric Psychiatry, 18,* 1088–1094.

Breitbart, W., Gibson, C., Poppito, S., & Berg, A., (2004). Psychotherapeutic interventions at the end of life: A focus on meaning and spirituality. *Canadian Journal of Psychiatry, 49*(6), 366–372.

Burnside, I., & Haight, B. K. (1992). Reminiscence and life review: Analysing each concept. *Journal of Advanced Nursing, 17*(7), 855–862.

Butler, R. (1963). The life review: An interpretation of reminiscence in the aged. *Psychiatry, 26,* 65–76.

Butler, R. (1974). Successful aging and the role of life review. *Journal of the American Geriatrics Society, 22,* 529–535.

Byock, I. (2004). *The four things that matter most: A book about living.* New York: Free Press.

Chiang, K. (2008). Evaluation of the effect of a life review group program on self-esteem and life satisfaction in the elderly. *International Journal of Geriatric Psychiatry, 23,* 7–10.

Chochinov, H. M., Hack, T., Hassard, T., Kristjanson, L. J., McClement, S., & Harlos, M. (2005). Dignity therapy: A novel psychotherapeutic intervention for patients near the end of life. *Journal of Clinical Oncology, 23,* 5520–5525.

Doka, K. J. (1993). *Living with life-threatening illness: A guide for patients, their families, and caregivers.* San Francisco: Jossey-Bass Publishers.

Erikson, E. H. (1959). *Identity and the life cycle.* New York: International Universities Press.

Erikson, E. H. (1963). *Childhood and society* (2nd ed.). New York: Norton.

Erlin, J., Mellors, M., Sereika, S., & Cook C. (2001). The use of life review to enhance quality of life of people living with AIDS: A feasibility study. *Quality of Life Research, 10,* 453–464.

Garland, J., & Garland, C. (2001). *Life review in health and social care.* Philadelphia: Taylor & Francis.

Graybeal, A., Sexton, J. D., & Pennebaker, J. W. (2002). The role of story-making in disclosure writing: The psychometrics of narrative. *Psychology and Health, 17,* 571–581.

Haber, D. (2006). Life review: Implementation, theory, research, and therapy. *International Journal of Aging and Human Development, 63*(2), 153–171.

Haight, B. K, & Davis, J. K. (1992). Examining key variables in selected reminiscing modalities. *International Psychogeriatrics, 4,* 279–290.

Haight, B., Michel Y., & Hendrix S. (1998). Life review: Preventing despair in newly relocated nursing home residents—short- and long-term effects. *International Journal of Aging and Human Development, 47,* 119–142.

Haight, B. K., Bachman, D. L., Hendrix, S., Wagner, M. T., Meeks, A., & Johnson, J. (2003). Life review: Treating the dyadic family unit with dementia. *Clinical Psychology and Psychotherapy, 10,* 165–174.

Hunter, E. G. (2007–2008). Beyond death: Inheriting the past and giving to the future, transmitting the legacy of one's self. *Omega: Journal of Death & Dying, 56*(4), 313–329.

Hunter, E. G., & Rowles, G. D. (2005). Leaving a legacy: Toward a typology. *Journal of Aging Studies, 19*(3), 327–347.

Jenko, M., Gonzalez, L., & Alley, P. (2010). Life review in critical care: Possibilities at the end of life. *Critical Care Nurse, 30*(1), 17–27.

Johnson, L. S. (2003). Facilitating spiritual meaning-making for the individual with a diagnosis of a terminal illness. *Counseling and Values, 47.*

Kartman, L. (1991). Life review: One aspect of making meaningful music for the elderly. *Activities, Adaptation & Aging, 15,* 45–52.

Klass, D., & Silverman, P. R. (1996). Introduction: What's the problem?. In D. Klass, P. R. Silverman, & S. L. Nickman (Eds.), *Continuing bonds: New understandings of grief* (pp. 3–27). Philadelphia: Taylor & Francis.

Lawler, K., Younger, J., Piferi, R., Jobe, R., Edmonson, K., & Jones, W. (2005). The unique effects of forgiveness on health: An exploration of pathways. *Journal of Behavioral Medicine, 28,* 157–167.

Lifton, R. J. (1979). *The broken connection: On death and the continuity of life.* New York: Simon & Schuster.

McAdams, D. P. (1993). *The stories we live by: Personal myths and the making of the self.* New York: William Morrow & Company.

McAdams, D. P. (2006). The role of narrative in personality psychology today. *Narrative Inquiry, 16*(1), 11–18.

McClement, S., Chochinov, H. M., Hack, T., Hassard, T., Kristjanson, L. J., & Harlos, M. (2007). Dignity therapy: Family member perspectives. *Journal of Palliative Medicine, 10*(5), 1076–1082.

Miller, M.(2009, April). *Harvard mental health letter.* Boston: Harvard Heath Publications.

Otis-Green, S. (2003). Legacy building. *Smith College Studies in Social Work, 73*(3), 395–404.

Pennebaker, J. W., & Seagal J. D. (1999). Forming a story: The health benefits of narrative. *Journal of Clinical Psychology, 55,* 1243–1254.

Puchalski, C., Ferrell, B., Virani, R., Otis-Green, S., Baird, P., Bull, J.,… Sulmasy, D. (2009). Improving the quality of spiritual care as a dimension of palliative care: The report of the consensus conference. *Journal of Palliative Medicine, 12*(10), 885–904.

Sadavoy J., & Lazarus L. (2000). Individual psychotherapy. In B. J. Sadock & V. A. Sadock (Eds.), *Comprehensive textbook of psychiatry* (7th ed.). Philadelphia: Lippincott Williams & Wilkins.

Serrano, J. P., Latorre, J. M., Gatz, M., & Montanes, J. (2004). Life review therapy using autobiographical retrieval practice for older adults with depressive symptomatology. *Psychology and Aging, 19*(2), 272–277.

Sherman, E. (1991). *Reminiscence and the self in old age.* New York: Springer Publishing Company.

Sherman, E. (1995). Reminiscentia: Cherished objects as memorabilia in late-life reminiscence. In J. Hendricks (Ed.), *The meaning of reminiscence and life review* (pp. 193–204). Amityville, NY: Baywood Publishing.

Silverman, P. R. & Nickman, S. L. (1996). Children's construction of their dead parents. In D. Klass, P. R. Silverman, & S. L. Nickman (Eds.), *Continuing bonds: New understandings of grief* (pp. 73–86). Philadelphia: Taylor & Francis.

Steinhauser, K. E., Alexander, S. C., Byock, I. R., George, L. K., Olsen, M. K., & Tulsky, J. A. (2008). Do preparation and life completion discussions improve functioning and quality of life in seriously ill patients? Pilot randomized control trial. *Journal of Palliative Medicine, 11*(9), 1234–1240.

Tyson-Rawson, K. (1996). Relationship and heritage: Manifestations of ongoing attachment following father death. In D. Klass, P. R. Silverman, & S. L. Nickman (Eds.), *Continuing bonds: New understandings of grief* (pp. 125–145). Philadelphia: Taylor & Francis.

Wallace, J. B. (1992). Reconsidering the life review: The social construction of talk about the past. *Gerontologist, 32*, 120–125.

Weiss, J. (1995). Cognitive therapy and life review therapy: Theoretical and therapeutic implications for mental health counselors. *Journal of Mental Health, 17*, 157–171.

Worden, W. J. (2002). *Grief counseling and grief therapy : A handbook for the mental health practitioner* (3rd ed.). New York: Springer Publications.

Yalom, I. D. (1980). *Existential psychotherapy.* New York: Basic Books.

CHAPTER 7

A Transdisciplinary Approach to Spiritual Care

Linda F. Piotrowski

Transdisciplinary health care involves reaching into the spaces between the disciplines to create positive health outcomes through collaboration. This model of care effectively integrates clinicians such as physicians, nurses, social workers, physical therapists, complementary and alternative medicine practitioners, physician assistants, community health workers, and other healthcare providers to create a team that provides comprehensive preventative primary care (Kilgo, Aldridge, & Denton, 2003).

Transdisciplinary care advocates call for broadening our notion of primary care to include a team working together to alleviate the burdens borne by patients with multiple co-morbidities and extenuating social circumstances (Ruddy & Rhee, 2005).

Most clinicians are trained to work in a medical setting within systems where acute needs are dealt with through mostly medical interventions. Today's healthcare system is moving toward the provision of bio-psychosocial-spiritual care.

Transdisciplinary palliative care is care that involves a team of care providers. In many acute care hospitals, a written consult request initiated by a patient's attending physician is required before a transdisciplinary palliative care team becomes involved in patient care. Once a consult request is received, the palliative care team begins their work.

The goal of palliative care as defined by the National Consensus Project for Quality Palliative Care (NCP) is:

> ...to prevent and relieve suffering and to support the best possible quality of life for patients and their families, regardless of the stage of disease or the need for other therapies.... Leadership, collaboration, coordination, and communication are key elements for effective integration of these disciplines and services. (NCP, 2009, p. 6)

> Spiritual and existential dimensions are assessed and responded to based upon the best available evidence, which is skillfully and systematically applied. (p. 49)

For many—indeed one could argue, for all—patients and their family members, this means the inclusion of attention to the spiritual as a part of their care. In order to tend to the spiritual nature of a person, one must make a distinction between religion and spirituality.

> Spirituality refers to an individual's or a group's relationship to the transcendent, however that may be construed. Spirituality is about the search for transcendent meaning. Most people express their spirituality in religious practice. Others express their spirituality exclusively in their relationships with nature, music, the arts, or a set of philosophical beliefs or relationships with friends and family. Religion on the other hand, is a set of beliefs, practices and language that characterizes a community that is searching for transcendent meaning in a particular way, generally on the basis of belief in a deity. Thus, although not everyone has a religion, everyone who searches for ultimate or transcendent meaning can be said to have spirituality. (Sulmasy, 2002, p. 25)

In February, 2009, a Consensus Project sponsored by the Archstone Foundation of Long Beach, California, was held in Pasadena, California. The goal of the conference was to identify points of agreement about spirituality as it applies to health care and to make recommendations to advance the delivery of quality spiritual care in palliative care. The consensus group agreed upon this definition of spirituality within the context of a healthcare environment: "Spirituality is the aspect of humanity that refers to the way individuals seek and express meaning and purpose and the way they experience their connectedness to the moment, to self, to others, to nature, and to the significant or sacred" (Puchalski et al., 2009, p. 887).

Additional recommendations from the Consensus Project on Improving the Quality of Spiritual Care as a Dimension of Palliative Care are as follows:
1. Spiritual care should be integral to a compassionate and patient-centered healthcare system model of care. Spiritual care models should be based on honoring the dignity of all people and on providing compassionate care.

2. Spiritual distress or religious struggle should be treated with the same intent and urgency as treatment for pain or any other medical or social problem.
3. Spirituality should be considered a patient vital sign. Just as pain is screened routinely, so should spiritual issues be a part of routine care. Institutional policies for spiritual history and screening must be integrated into intake policies and ongoing assessment of care.
4. Spiritual care models should be interdisciplinary, and clinical settings should have a Clinical Pastoral Education-trained board-certified chaplain as part of the interprofessional team. The spiritual care member of the palliative care team is ideally a board-certified chaplain. (Puchalski et al., 2009, p. 891)

Religious community and spiritual practices are important aspects of the lives of a substantial portion of the U.S. population. According to a Gallup Poll, approximately 70% of Americans are members of a church or synagogue and 82% of adults consider religion "very important" to themselves. Eighty percent indicate that they use prayer in times of crisis and 95% of those believe that their prayers are answered. These rates of religious interest have remained fairly constant in the United States from the mid-1960s through the 1990s (Gallup & Lindsay, 1999; Weaver, Koenig, & Flannelly, 2008, p. 92).

The chaplain on a transdisciplinary team fills many roles. The chaplain's primary responsibility to the patient is to complete a spiritual assessment, ensuring that the spiritual and religious needs of the patient and family are addressed. Assessing a patient's spiritual needs is the way in which the chaplain can then fulfill other roles as advocate, educator, and coordinator.

With spiritual assessment completed, the chaplain becomes the patient's spiritual advocate, claiming a place at the healthcare table. With the transdisciplinary team, the chaplain assists in the development of a comprehensive care plan that acknowledges and incorporates the patient's spiritual needs.

Education related to spirituality and religion and their role in patient care is the chaplain's ongoing responsibility. It takes place through formal educational presentations throughout the institution and informally through interactions at the patient bedside and in transdisciplinary team meetings. Creating an awareness of the spiritual and training other team members to screen for patients' spiritual needs and the necessity of referrals are critical components of the ongoing education provided by the chaplain team member.

The chaplain's responsibility to educate extends beyond the walls of the institution. According to Jacobs (2010), chaplains can engage with community clergy to partner in caring for the spiritual needs of patients. She writes,

> Professional chaplains, for the most part, focus not only on what is happening inside that institution's walls, but also know the value of reaching out to clergy in the surrounding communities. Workshops, conversations, discussion groups and filling in for a clergy person in the pulpit are just some of the ways that chaplains interact with local clergy. Chaplains can help clergy navigate the sometimes difficult to understand culture of a hospital, and can assist with educating congregations about advance directives, hospital etiquette, options available for hospice, long-term care facilities and so on. (p. 14)

Once a spiritual assessment is completed and a care plan is developed, the chaplain engages the patient in addressing their spiritual needs. At this point, it is critical to determine along with the patient the level of involvement the patient desires on the part of their personal faith community. If the patient is not a member of a faith community, it is important to explore their desire to become a part of a community.

Individuals rely on their faith communities as a place to gather with people who hold similar beliefs about God, the nature of life and death, and how to worship. On nearly a weekly basis, people gather to celebrate new life through initiation rituals and mourn deaths through funerals, memorial services, and other rituals. The faith community is no stranger to illness, grief, and loss. In his letter from the editor's desk, Buchanan (2010) describes the reaction of Elaine Pagles, not a churchgoer, to recently delivered news that her 2-year-old son was critically ill:

> Standing in the back of that church, I recognized, uncomfortably, that I needed to be there…. Here was a place to weep without imposing tears upon your child; and here was a heterogeneous community that had gathered to sing, to celebrate, to acknowledge common needs, and to deal with what we cannot control or imagine…. Here is a family that knows how to face death.

...The rock bottom reason for the church's existence is to be a community that knows how to deal with death. Indeed, spiritual communities are gathering places for the sorrowful and those who mourn. (p. 3)

Faith communities provide support in a number of ways. Congregational care and support are often expressed in practical ways such as provision of babysitting services, meals, and rides to medical appointments. Support is offered through worship opportunities, whether in the traditional place of worship (church, synagogue, temple) or through home visitation programs where trained volunteers bring sacraments, prayer, and the comfort of companionship. Faith communities are ever more aware of accommodating the needs of the ill and elderly in their worship places in order to alleviate the sense of isolation and loneliness often felt by church members unable to participate in services due to disability.

Pastors, rabbis, imams, and other faith leaders can utilize the natural rhythm of worship and sacred scriptures to assist their congregants in becoming more comfortable talking about issues of illness, healing, death, and dying.

A faith community's care extends beyond the experience of illness to assistance with planning for funeral and memorial services. Funeral choirs, volunteers who will prepare a funeral breakfast or brunch, even volunteers to remain at the family home to care for pets are among the services congregations offer. Care does not end with funeral or memorial services. Often congregations sponsor grief and loss support groups for members. Increasingly, these groups are becoming interfaith, offering companionship and a place to explore the challenges of grief and loss within a caring and supportive community.

A CASE STUDY

Returning to the hospital setting, we meet Marian, a 43-year-old mother of three children (ages 8, 12, and 20) with a malignant brain tumor that has not responded to treatment. In spite of her diagnosis, Marian had been able to fulfill most of her activities of daily life, including her work as a bookkeeper. Marian was then hospitalized for intractable pain. She and her husband James, a welder, struggled. They joked that it was a good thing that the economy was so bad and that he was laid off from his work as it provided him the time to care for the children while

Marian was incapacitated. In spite of their attempts at humor, the future looked bleak to them. Since Marian was then unable to work, they worried about how the bills would be paid. Their children were aware of Marian's health problems but did not know the extent of her illness. As parents, they worried about the impact her advancing disease would have on them.

On their initial visit to Marian, the palliative care team's attending physician, nurse practitioner, and varied members of the team introduced themselves, explaining their role in her care. They proceeded to inquire about Marian's level of pain and other symptoms, and assured her that they will do their best to assist her in making them manageable. They mentioned other members of the team and the services they could provide. (Depending upon the setting, other team members might include the social worker, healing arts practitioners, a board-certified chaplain, volunteer visitors, and others.) Having addressed her pain and disease symptoms, the palliative care team members talked with Marian about other aspects of her life, including her goals for her care. Their intake assessment was comprehensive, including her physical, social, spiritual, and psychological needs.

When the transdisciplinary team gathered to plan for Marian's care, the chaplain noted that Marian and her husband spoke of being affiliated with a faith community and that this might be a source of additional support for the patient and family as they face the progression of Marian's disease.

Upon visiting Marian, the chaplain discovered that Marian and her husband were very private people. They had worked hard to keep others in their community unaware of the severity of Marian's disease. Over the course of several visits, the chaplain worked with Marian and James around spiritual issues including faith, God's role in illness, hope, fear of the future, concern for Marian's children, and her legacy. They also acknowledged the impact Marian's disease was having on her family and the possible benefits that might result by inviting other people into her circle of care. The chaplain gently introduced the idea of inviting Marian's pastor into this conversation in order to have ongoing spiritual support once she returned to her home. Once Marian and James gave permission to contact their pastor, the chaplain contacted her and invited her to the hospital to meet with Marian and James. Together, they explored Marian and James's spiritual needs. They determined how to proceed with involving the pastor and their faith community in Marian's ongoing care.

As Marian's disease progressed, their pastor visited on a weekly basis. She was able to assist Marian in creating an ethical will in which Marian was able to express her hopes and dreams for her children. Together, they created letters for each one of the children to be given to them on various significant occasions in the coming years. Their pastor was able to facilitate meaningful conversations between James and Marian in which they explored their hopes and dreams, fears and grief.

As Marian's condition worsened, their pastor was able to gently invite Marian and James to open up the circle of people who had knowledge of Marian's condition. They gave permission for their pastor to include them in the church's weekly worship services and to ask church members for help with their practical needs.

Hospice was engaged for Marian's care. With Marian and James's permission, their pastor invited a few members of the congregation to assist James with the responsibilities related to the care of the house and the children. The volunteers took on tasks of housecleaning, laundry, and the preparation of healthy meals, freeing James to spend time with Marian and their children.

With their pastor's assistance, Marian was able to express her wishes regarding her funeral and burial service. Marian dictated a message to be read during the service. With her pastor, Marian chose readings and hymns that were meaningful to her and her family.

Marian died with James and her children at her bedside. Shortly after her death, James called her pastor. Their pastor came and supported James and the children in their grief. She helped him contact the hospice nurse, who arrived and helped with practical details. The pastor was a calming presence—remaining with James and the children well into the night.

In the following days, the funeral service was celebrated according to Marian's plans and desires. The congregation assisted with everything from the singing at the service to the funeral breakfast to supplying meals for the family for weeks after Marian's death. As weeks turned into months, Marian and James's pastor met with James to talk about life without Marian. The congregation, weekly worship, and a local support group became a safe place for James and the children to mourn.

A loving and caring congregation supported Marian and James. This support was made possible in part by the inclusion of their spiritual needs in the plan of care developed by the transdisciplinary team at their hospital. It was also made possible by the work of a pastor who was unafraid to invite her congregation to make their faith and love visible by acts of generosity and caring. While not all congregations and clergy are as comfortable with illness, the dying process, and death itself as Marian's was, most all are eager to learn how to be a welcoming place where the sorrowing can find comfort and support.

Various resources are available for faith congregations to learn how to support members in times of illness, dying, and death. Three helpful resources are:

- "It's About How You LIVE—In Faith," available free of charge from Caring Connections, an initiative of the National Hospice and Palliative Care Organization (NHPCO, 2008)
- "The Unbroken Circle: A Toolkit for Congregations Around Illness, End of Life and Grief," by James L. Brooks (2009)
- "State-wide Hospice Clergy End-of-Life Education Enhancement Project," available free of charge from Hospice Foundation of America at www.hospicefoundation.org

One of the cornerstones of philosophical anthropology is that human beings are intrinsically spiritual. This is based on the notion of the human person as a being in relationships. Sickness, rightly understood, is a disruption of right relationships (Sulmasy, 2002, p. 26).

By advocating for patients' spiritual needs, assisting patients in making connections with faith communities, educating transdisciplinary team members, and alerting religious leaders and congregations to the critical role they can play in supporting patients and families in times of serious illness, death, and dying, the chaplain on the transdisciplinary team ensures that the patient and family receive the best care possible.

Linda F. Piotrowski, MTS, BCC, is a board-certified chaplain through the National Association of Catholic Chaplains. She holds a masters of theology from St. Francis Seminary in Milwaukee, Wisconsin. Additionally, she was educated in the Center to Advance Palliative Care programs and completed the Metta Institute's Compassionate Care for the Dying Training. A chaplain for 23 years, Ms. Piotrowski has ministered in acute and long-term care, home hospice, and parish and congregational settings. A member of the Dartmouth-Hitchcock Medical Center's chaplaincy department, she currently ministers as the pastoral care coordinator and chaplain for the palliative care and oncology services at Dartmouth Hitchcock Medical Center and the Norris Cotton Cancer Center in Lebanon, New Hampshire.

REFERENCES

Brooks, J. L. (2009). *The unbroken circle: A toolkit for congregations around illness, end of life and grief.* Durham, NC: Duke Institute on Care at the End of Life.

Buchanan, J. (2010). A place to mourn. *The Christian Century, 10*(12), 3.

Gallup, G., & Lindsay, M. D. (1999). *Surveying the religious landscape: Trends in U.S. beliefs.* Harrisburg, PA: Morehouse Publishing.

Jacobs, M. (2010). Speaking of dying. *Healing Spirit, 5*(1) 12–14.

Kilgo, J. L., Aldridge, J., & Denton, B. (2003). Transdisciplinary teaming: A vital component of inclusive services. *Focus on inclusive education, 1*(1). Available at http://www.udel.edu/bateman/acei/inclusivefall03.htm

National Consensus Project for Quality Palliative Care. (2009). *Clinical practice guidelines for quality palliative care* (2nd ed.). Pittsburgh, PA: National Consensus Project.

National Hospice and Palliative Care Organization. (2008, August 21). *"It's about how you LIVE—in faith"—new resources enhance hospice community's support for spiritual care* [Press Release]. Retrieved from http://www.nhpco. org/i4a/pages/index.cfm?pageid=5705

Puchalski, C., Ferrell, B., Virani, R., Otis-Green, S., Baird, P., Bull, J.,...
Sulmasy, D. (2009). Improving the quality of spiritual care as a dimension of
palliative care: The report of the consensus conference. *Journal of Palliative
Medicine, 12*(10), 885–904.

Ruddy, G., & Rhee, K. (2005). Transdisciplinary teams in primary care for
the underserved: A literature review. *Journal of Health Care for the Poor and
Underserved, 16*(2), 248–256.

Sulmasy, D. (2002). A biopsychosocial-spiritual model for the care of patients
at the end of life. *The Gerontologist, 42*, Special Issue III, 24–33.

Weaver, A. J., Koenig, H. G., & Flannelly, L. T. (2008). Nurses and chaplains:
Natural allies. *Journal of Health Care Chaplaincy, 14*(2), 91–98.

Spiritual Needs and Nursing Care

Reinette Powers Murray

Research suggests that some nurses do not feel adequately prepared to meet their patients' spiritual needs; do not fully understand the concept of spiritual care; are not comfortable with their own meaning of spirituality; or do not have the time in their daily practice to approach the subject with their patients. Results from previous studies have shown a range in nurses' definitions of *spirituality* and feelings about sharing their beliefs with their patients (Pulchaski, 2004). These studies show that registered nurses are not comfortable addressing spirituality with their patients and have increased awareness of the need to understand the very concept of spirituality.

HISTORY OF SPIRITUALITY AND MEDICINE

Spirituality has been linked to medicine and healing for centuries, as evidenced by the Native American medicine man, the shaman, and various religious healing practices. However, in the 20th century, modern medicine has focused more on the disease process while leaving the spiritual and religious issues related to the act of dying to the hospital pastoral care team or patients' personal ministers or priests. The history of Western medicine is one of gradual (and now virtually complete) disengagement from religious or spiritual explanations of disease and cure for an almost total embrace of biological explanations of disease along with technologically sophisticated treatments.

NECESSITY FOR NURSES PROVIDING SPIRITUAL CARE

Despite multiple studies that demonstrate the necessity of fulfilling spiritual care needs, patients continue to approach the end-of-life experience without having their spiritual care needs addressed. Historically, the literature tended to describe nursing as a *calling* or *vocation,* which included a spiritual dimension or commitment. Florence Nightingale considered her work more than a job; she considered it a vocation.

Today, nursing research increasingly claims an ethical responsibility to provide spiritual care. In recognition of the spiritual needs of patients, the Joint Commission on Accreditation of Healthcare Organizations (2002) stated, "Patients have a fundamental right to considerate care that safeguards their personal dignity and respects their psychological needs, culture, and spiritual values" (p. R1-15). However, nursing is currently viewed as more of a socioeconomic stepladder and more nurses have stepped away from the spiritual values that were part of the profession at its inception.

BARRIERS TO ADDRESSING SPIRITUAL NEEDS

Multiple research studies addressing patient's spiritual needs at the end of life show that many nurses do not feel comfortable addressing the topic with their patients or clients. Is this problem due to nurses' personal uncertainty about what spirituality is, or rather, the lack of education in nursing programs regarding spiritual care needs?

Pesut (2003) states that members of the profession increasingly refer to the necessity of spiritual nursing and even support the ethical nature of spiritual necessity. However, positions on spirituality are often contradictory when conceptualizing spirituality. Pesut advises that the focus should be on understanding and incorporating multiple characterizations of spirituality in society and then continuing to promote dialogue.

EDUCATION NEEDS IN PROVIDING SPIRITUAL CARE TOOLS FOR NURSES

According to a study completed by Catanzaro (2006), there is a serious discontinuity today between the nursing profession's standards of practice—requiring nurses to address the spiritual needs of clients—and nursing curricula, which do not consistently prepare students to address the spiritual needs of clients. Can or should nurses be expected to address spiritual concerns with their patients if the concepts or dimensions of spiritual care have not been addressed in their nursing curriculum? How can nursing education programs incorporate spirituality teaching into their curricula?

Pesut (2003) states that, although many nursing education programs are searching for ways to incorporate spirituality into the curriculum, it remains a point of debate how this should be done. A study conducted by the American Association of Colleges of Nursing (AACN) recommends that nurse education programs should ensure that nurses can comprehend the meaning of human spirituality and recognize its relationship with culture, behavior, health, and healing, and then be able to plan and implement appropriate spiritual care. As nursing professionals explore their own sense of purpose and spirituality and discover what gives life meaning, they will become better able to understand and relate to patients.

Reinette Powers Murray, MSN, CNS, RN, is owner of The Peaceful Journey End-of-Life Process Program. She also is certified as a Train-the-Trainer for End-of-Life Nursing Education (ELNEC). She has worked as an assistant professor of nursing at the university level, caring for patients with students and demonstrating spiritual care assessment to nursing students. Mrs. Murray has published spirituality research in the Journal of Hospice and Palliative Care, *presented her research at the a National Hospice and Palliative Care conference, and is currently working on her doctorate in nursing practice with a focus on the need for spirituality education for nurses and its inclusion in nursing programs. She is certified to provide End-of-Life Nursing Education Consortium (ELNEC) education to healthcare professionals.*

REFERENCES

American Association of Colleges of Nursing (1986). *Essentials of college and university education for professional nursing.* Washington, DC: American Association of Colleges of Nursing.

Catanzaro, A. (2006). The meaning and place of spirituality in the education of student nurses from the mid-1800's to the twenty-first century. *Eastern Nursing Research Society.* Retrieved from http:/enrs.confex.com/enrs/18am/techprogram/P1589.htm

Joint Commission on Accreditation of Healthcare Organizations. (2002). *Patient rights and practice.* Retrieved January 21, 2005, from http://www.jcaho.org/standard/camhen_obs.html

Puchalski, C. (2004). A spiritual history. *Supportive Voice, 5*(3), 12–13.

CHAPTER 8

Spiritual Care:
An Organizational Perspective

Richard B. Fife

Who is there in all the world who listens to us? Here I am—this is me in my nakedness, with my wounds, my secret grief, my despair, my betrayal, my pain which I can't express, my terror, my abandonment. Oh, listen to me for a day, an hour, a moment, lest I expire in my terrible wilderness, my lonely silence. Oh God is there no one to listen?

Seneca (quoted in Saunders, 1988)

FOUNDATION OF SPIRITUAL CARE IN HOSPICE

In the opening section of the National Hospice and Palliative Care Organization's (NHPCO) *Guidelines for Spiritual Care in Hospice,* the authors state, "The historical roots of the hospice movement are deeply imbedded in the soil of spiritually motivated service. In Europe, care for the dying sprang from religious faith and was characterized by a sense of divine calling" (NHPCO, 2009, p. *i*). However, this may be something of an overstatement. First of all, it is a stretch to call what happened in early Europe really *spiritual* in nature; second, it is difficult to connect this to the present day hospice movement.

During the 11th and 12th centuries, there were monasteries throughout Europe before most of them would be broken up by the Reformation. These were religious communities that did indeed provide shelter and a place to rest for weary travelers. Most of these travelers were men involved in the Crusades and were simply helped with their physical needs and then went on their way (Farleigh Hospice, 2008). For the most part, they were not terminally ill persons given a place of comfort as they were dying. The use of the word *hospice* may be correct here but it does not necessarily refer to the dying. The word itself comes from the Latin *hospis* meaning "host and a guest" (Farleigh Hospice, 2008). It developed into *hospitality* as its intended meaning. Perhaps one derives the spiritual foundation from the fact that the hosts were primarily monasteries, but then one also must recognize the widespread religious influence throughout Europe during this period. One must also ask if the emphasis may have been on the *religious* as opposed to the *spiritual.*

The word *hospice* was not used to describe a place where the terminally ill were looked after until the 19th century. In France, Ireland, and England, there were religious communities that took care of those who were considered incurable (Farleigh Hospice, 2008). Again, one connects the spiritual with the religious partially due to the nature of the communities that cared for the dying. However, one must also consider the limitations of medical practice at the time and ask exactly what could be done to control pain and relieve symptoms. Indeed, not until the discovery of penicillin and other such medications in the 20th century could one hope to control simple infections. Therefore, the emphasis had to be on simply providing a home for the incurables.

This is not to say that there was no foundation for spiritual care in what could be considered hospice during these periods. After all, rest and peace could be found in these places for many and this could also perhaps be seen as refreshment for the soul. Furthermore, the religious communities could conceivably help one to at least question the meaning of one's life. But the real spiritual foundation of hospice awaited a period when there was a sharp distinction between religious and secular and there was the potential to control symptoms of physical pain, thus allowing reflection and action on spiritual needs.

The modern hospice movement that began in the 1950s and 1960s can be honestly labeled as *spiritual* because a new view of dying began to emerge that took into account things such as meaning and dignity. Previous to this time, there had been a passive approach to caring for the dying. Now there was a more focused awareness on the total suffering of the dying and their physical and mental condition. This awareness was made manifest most strongly in the work of Cicely Saunders at St. Joseph's Hospice in London. In a systematic and well-organized way, she listened to patients' stories of illness and suffering and developed the concept of *total pain* (Saunders, 1988). She definitely was concerned about pain management as indicated in her message, "Constant pain needs constant control" (Saunders, 1960). To her, pain management was not just the physical but also the spiritual and emotional. This is reflected in the patient who said to her, "All of me is wrong" (Saunders, 1964). The success at St. Joseph's, the work of Cicely Saunders, and how an excellent model of care came out of this situation forms the real spiritual foundation of hospice care.

TRYING TO DEFINE EXCELLENT SPIRITUAL CARE

Spiritual care in hospice is a shared responsibility and concerns all of the various disciplines. (NHPCO, 2009, p. 5)

While all members of the hospice team touch the spiritual lives of patients, the spiritual counselor is that team member whose professional expertise is spiritual care. (NHPCO, 2009, p. 6)

Spirituality is that part of each individual which longs for meaning, integrity, beauty, dignity, love and acceptance. (VITAS Concept of Spirituality)

The author's immediate background is almost 30 years of experience with VITAS Healthcare Corporation, one of the largest hospice companies in the United States. From its beginning, VITAS recognized the role of the chaplain in the interdisciplinary team and the hospice itself. Federal regulations never mandated that there be a chaplain on every team or even that each hospice have its own chaplain. Some examples of federal regulations regarding spiritual care in hospice follow:

- "[Spiritual] counseling services must be available to both the individual and the family" (United States Code of Federal Regulation [C.F.R.] 418.88).
- "Counseling, including pastoral counseling is available on a 24-hour basis" (C.F.R. 418.70).
- A plan of care "is a complete assessment of the patient's and family needs which include their spiritual status" (C.F.R. 418.68).
- The hospice "has an interdisciplinary team that includes a pastor or other counselor" (C.F.R. 418.68).

These federal regulations could actually be fulfilled by part-time clergy, contracted spiritual counselors, or community volunteer clergy. What set VITAS apart at its very beginning was its insistence that every team have a chaplain. Part of the reason for this focus was that one of its founders, Hugh Westbrook, was a clergyperson himself. He insisted on the importance of spiritual care in the VITAS hospice community and saw the chaplain as the person directly responsible for coordinating the spiritual care in the team and the hospice. Therefore, the first tenet of good spiritual care in VITAS was an actual commitment to spiritual care. It would be a commitment that would extend to patients, families, staff, and the community. Although the person most directly responsible for excellent spiritual care in hospice is the spiritual counselor, every member of the team provides spiritual care. To better understand this, one needs to separate the *religious* from the *spiritual*. VITAS believes that while every person is not necessarily religious, at some level all people are spiritual. The religious may involve rituals, belief systems, and spiritual dynamics. These things may necessitate the presence of a chaplain or clergyperson, at least to the patient or family member. Part of the role of the chaplain in VITAS is to deal with these religious matters and to help the team members to deal with the spiritual questions as they arise.

The spiritual needs of patients and families recognized over the years by VITAS are the need for meaning; the need for hope; the need for love and acceptance; the need for dignity; and the need for a sense of an ultimate spiritual source.

Meaning

Meaning can be very subjective and difficult to define and it will vary from patient to patient. Some patients find meaning in ordinary tasks completed on a regular basis. Others look for meaning to give life a sense of worth or to understand what one may be enduring. Even in the midst of great suffering and terrible events, one continues to search for some type of meaning. Two examples come to mind. The first is expressed in the biblical book of Job. A series of terrible events befall Job that ravages all that he has. The events— human-caused and nonhuman—take their toll on Job and his family. Even Job's wife urges him to curse God and die. But Job finds meaning even in chaos and great suffering. "[Job] still maintains his integrity, though you [Satan] incited me against him to ruin him without any reason" (Job 2:3, New International Version). The second example is more modern and yet similar in many ways. Viktor Frankl was a psychiatrist in Germany under the rule of the Nazis. He was a prisoner in the concentration camp at Auschwitz, where he suffered greatly and saw his world crumble. However, he lived to write a book titled *Man's Search for Meaning*. One of his most famous statements from the book is "…he who knows the *why* of his existence will be able to bear almost any *how*" (Frankl, 1963, p. 127).

All of us want to make sense out of life. Often this need is heightened as one approaches death. The VITAS caregiver listens empathetically to the patient, without giving advice, allowing him or her to find their own meaning. The VITAS caregiver might ask the patient and family questions like, "Where do you find meaning? What difficulties do you have in understanding what is happening to you?"

Hope

Often it is hope that gives meaning to life. A hospice patient is, by definition, terminally ill. Many people would find no hope in a situation where life is so limited. Indeed, if a hospice patient had no real hope, he or she would find it difficult to live another day. But hope is very much alive—just not necessarily a hope for a cure. One patient's granddaughter was going to graduate from college in 8 months. She lived in the hope that she would see her granddaughter graduate. Another patient hoped he would see the sun rise again the next day, as it had so many times during his lifetime. The hospice patient needs hope just like every other living person. Here, the VITAS caregiver invites reflection by asking the patient, "What is it that you count upon during your illness?" or "In what ways has your hope changed during your illness?"

Love and Acceptance

Love and acceptance is a spiritual need patients have that reaches out to others or God. It is easy to feel unaccepted when one becomes ill. Friends often tend to neglect those who are dying. Here, the interdisciplinary team has a great responsibility to see that the patient is not neglected—that the patient feels love and acceptance. In the 1980s, soon after the beginning of the U.S. AIDS epidemic, VITAS created a hospice in Miami for the sole purpose of taking care of patients dying of AIDS-related illnesses. This was a period when society was frightened by AIDS, had little understanding of what was happening, and shunned those who were HIV positive. It was difficult to find a group of terminally ill patients more in need of love and acceptance. At one point, the VITAS hospice was taking care of over 250 AIDS patients a day. One of the greatest things the hospice caregivers had to offer was a sense of love and acceptance. For reflection, the VITAS caregiver might ask, "To what degree do you feel loved and valued by others?" or "Do you feel at peace with yourself?"

Dignity

The author walked into a pharmacy, placed some items to purchase on the counter, and when the salesperson looked up, tears came to her eyes. She was looking at the name on the shirt—VITAS—and she exclaimed, "My sister just died and you helped her to die with such dignity." The salesperson had many other things to say but she began with the word *dignity*. Like so many hospice patients, she recognized the spiritual need for a person to be treated as a human being. It is so important to be treated humanely. With hospice patients, this means to help them maintain their freedom and independence as much as possible. It means caregivers must be willing to be human with their patients, to see them as fellow human beings and not just as terminally ill patients. Here, the VITAS caregiver might ask the patient how illness has affected his or her sense of worth or if the patient feels respected and treated with dignity.

A Sense of an Ultimate Spiritual Source

Of the five spiritual needs recognized by VITAS caregivers, this one is somewhat more elusive. It may be God, nature, or some other meaningful source. Most patients have a need to be a part of something larger than themselves—something that gives meaning and purpose to life. It often helps to listen and VITAS trains its staff to ask questions to identify this spiritual need. This may include, What is your concept, if any, of God? To what degree does your belief in God help you cope during your illness or loss? Are you struggling to be in control of certain things? What would be helpful to let go of?

TWO ASSESSMENTS: SELF-ASSESSMENT AND SPIRITUAL ASSESSMENT

Self-Assessment

VITAS stresses the need for all team members providing care to be familiar with the important elements of their own spirituality and to identify personal spiritual biases. A few examples of the questions VITAS asks their team members to consider in their spiritual self-assessments include:

- What is your concept of spirituality?
- Are there aspects of your spirituality that you feel strongly about?
- Are there values which you feel others should have?
- How well do you work with patients and families whose spiritual values differ from your own?
- How do you consider yourself religious? In what ways?
- What makes you feel hopeful, respected, loved, accepted?
- What gives your life meaning and purpose?

Spiritual Assessment

The VITAS chaplain is the person who initiates and develops the spiritual assessment of each patient but the team members in contact with the patient and family provide valuable information for the process. The assessment is an ongoing instrument that begins at admission, goes on through the dying process, and continues into bereavement. The spiritual assessment in VITAS addresses spiritual pain, spiritual formation, and spiritual resolution. In what ways are the patient and family struggling with meaning, hope, acceptance, and dignity? Formation involves examining the spiritual patterns and beliefs of the patient and family and then identifying where these beliefs do not contribute to their ability to cope and detract from their quality of life. Resolution looks at the need for spiritual closure in which both religious and spiritual needs are examined.

In order to provide proper spiritual assessment and to effectively provide for the spiritual and religious needs of patients, family, and staff, VITAS recognizes that chaplains must be properly educated, trained, and certified. In general, VITAS follows the suggested standards of education, training, and other qualifications specified by the National Hospice and Palliative Care Organization. With more than 200 chaplains working for the company, VITAS also recognizes the need for continuing training. In response to this need, it hired Dr. Martha Rutland to develop a companywide Clinical Pastoral Education (CPE) program to be properly certified. To increase the quality of spiritual care that her groups provide, she ensured that care teams include not only chaplains, but also social workers, nurses, team leaders, and others. Her leadership has strengthened the role of the chaplain in the training of team members and has provided needed spiritual training for all members of the team. She has helped the chaplains, nurses, home health aides, and other team members to look at the broad themes surrounding terminally ill persons and to listen to what is really being said. In reality, these broad themes of meaning and life-review, the search for completion, the desire to not be a burden, and the need for symptom control have been well-documented by palliative care and hospice clinicians as central themes in conversations with the dying. VITAS has always recognized that the primary role of the caregiving team is to listen and support the patient and family without judgment. Listening, caring, and demonstrating empathy are perhaps the most important aspects of spiritual care that any team member or other individual can provide.

The spiritual person is not there
To be seen and heard, but
To see and to hear...
To be a part of a moment
When eyes and ears might open.
Juliette Jones

GUIDELINES FOR SPIRITUAL CARE IN HOSPICE

Hospice patients often ask the *why* questions: Why me? Why now? Why am I being punished? Why is God not with me? Why does God not take me? They may be asking for specific answers. VITAS trains the team to invite the person to talk about what he or she is experiencing. They tell the team members to listen rather than to give advice, to avoid answering tough questions, and to be nonjudgmental. The team member may simply say, "Tell me more about what you are feeling," or "It sounds like you've been struggling with this. Can you share what you are feeling?" The team member needs to respond to the spiritual distress of the patient or family member but must also recognize one's limitations in helping persons with their spiritual needs. VITAS trains team members to recognize spiritual distress through expressions of meaninglessness, anger, unresolved feelings, or difficulty in finding meaning in the midst of suffering.

VITAS instructors tell a simple story when training caregivers for spiritual care: Diane, a certified home health aide, had been visiting a patient for several months when the patient asked to receive communion, a Christian ritual, from a chaplain. "I had a church up North but haven't joined one since I moved to Florida." Because she sensed there might be a spiritual need involved in the request, Diane probed further. "You mentioned belonging to a church up North."

"Yes," the patient replied. "The thing I miss most is the sense of family and the friends I had at the church. I sure don't have that now. I really miss Pastor Jones. We were good friends." Diane continued to listen as the patient shared all that she missed. After they finished their conversation, she called the team chaplain and mentioned the request for communion. She also shared the patient's need for a sense of belonging and friendship and that she missed her church and pastor. The chaplain thanked Diane not only for helping to identify the patient's spiritual needs in addition to her religious needs, but also for providing spiritual support by listening and conveying empathy.

SPIRITUAL CARE: AN ORGANIZATIONAL PERSPECTIVE

To provide effective spiritual care and meet the spiritual needs of patients and families, the following items are important:

- The hospice must have a strong commitment to providing spiritual care.
- The hospice needs to develop comprehensive policies and procedures for the spiritual care of patients and families.
- The hospice needs to recruit qualified chaplains to be ultimately responsible for spiritual care.

- Chaplains should receive continuous training, whether CPE or other workshops.
- Team members need to understand "spiritual needs"—meaning, hope, love and acceptance, dignity, and the need for an ultimate spiritual source.
- All team members need to do a personal assessment of their own beliefs and values.
- Team members need to be trained about spiritual needs and a variety of belief systems.
- Chaplains, aided by team members, need to develop a spiritual assessment and a plan of care for patients.
- Team members need to be trained in how to be sensitive to questions relating to spiritual needs.
- Team members need to know how best to introduce patients to the chaplain.
- Last, but certainly not least, in order to even hear the spiritual needs of hospice patients, the organization must have an effective program for pain management.

Key to providing effective spiritual care is having a person or persons designated and fully qualified to fill the role of trainer and teacher in this area. All hospice staff—nurses, home health aides, social workers, physicians, volunteers, as well as chaplains—have a role in providing spiritual care. However, if someone does not take charge, it may not be done in an effective and professional manner. Furthermore, not just any clergyperson is comfortable with this task. In a study on spiritual care at the end of life conducted by the Missoula Demonstration Project, the researchers point out that many clergy lack training in end-of-life care (Byock, Norris, Strohmaier, & Asp, 2004). Doka and Jendreski suggest that clergy's lack of education about grief is an obstacle that prevents them from being of greater solace to the bereaved (1985). In his book, *The Dying Soul*, Mark Cobb makes clear that it takes more than a cursory inclusion of spiritual needs in a nursing care model or a hope that people will absorb spiritual insight in the course of their daily care (Cobb, 2001). Cobb states that people's desire for spiritual support at the end of life is evident and argues that this support should be provided by trained professionals who have more than a vague understanding of theological, pastoral, and spiritual issues (Cobb, 2001). It cannot be overemphasized that for organizations and their team members to successfully provide excellent spiritual care, special care must be taken in selecting a spiritual coordinator, chaplain, or a series of chaplains for the task.

Problems for the Organization in Providing Spiritual Care

Paul Brenner points out that in 2001, about two-thirds of hospice patients die within 30 days of admission, making hospice much more oriented toward crisis management because death is imminent "rather than facilitating a thoughtful, intentional, progressive experience of the end of life that stresses its spiritual dimension and meaning" (Brenner, 2001). Simply put, there often is no time for the spiritual—even if you have the personnel trained for that purpose. How many times does one hear a hospice worker say that so much more could have been done to help the patient and family emotionally and spiritually if the patient had been admitted earlier?

A second problem for the organization relates to the shifting makeup of hospice patients and their families. At one time, virtually all hospice patients were white and middle class. This still tends to describe the majority. However, times are changing. NHPCO points this out in their *Guidelines for Spiritual Care in Hospice* (NHPCO, 2009). There is now a wide group of belief systems, cultures, and ethnic backgrounds that make up the hospice population. NHPCO says that "hospice spiritual counselors take a leading role in providing education to the interdisciplinary team...to serve persons of different backgrounds more compassionately and effectively" (p. 16). This means that the chaplain must continuously learn about various belief systems, customs, and practices and find a way to impart this knowledge to all team members. NHPCO (2009, p. 16) provides three additional guidelines for chaplains in this respect:

1. Hospice spiritual counselors support and advocate access to care for all patients and families facing terminal illness regardless of age, gender, nationality, race, creed, sexual orientation, disability, diagnosis, availability of a primary caregiver or ability to pay.

2. Spiritual counselors, community clergy and spiritual leaders and/or clergy from diverse linguistic, cultural and religious and spiritual backgrounds should be included on hospice staff in order to better address the linguistic, cultural and diverse spiritual needs of patients, families and staff.

3. Hospice spiritual counselors utilize community resources and establish relationships with the different cultural groups to heighten their awareness of beliefs, traditions, and practices that impact the delivery of hospice services.

These guidelines point out challenges to hospices trying to provide effective spiritual care. Not every hospice can provide chaplains for every team, chaplains that have been trained in CPE, chaplains that will be allowed the time to further their education on a continuous basis, chaplains that can represent various cultures and belief systems, or even chaplains that can adequately train other team members to provide spiritual care. In many cases one has to depend on community clergy and whatever printed resources may be available.

The chaplain may also meet most of the requirements for the hospice position, but he or she may too "religious," too "narrow," or not ecumenically oriented. It then becomes difficult for the chaplain to provide spiritual care to diverse populations or to properly train other team members in spiritual matters. Thus, it becomes very important for the organization to do proper recruiting and background research for potential chaplains.

A third challenge for providing spiritual care in the organization is the somewhat natural inclination to turn over all spiritual or religious concerns to the chaplain. The nurse, home health aide, or other team members may feel uncomfortable with spiritual questions and tell the patient, "We have a chaplain on the team that can help you with those questions. May I call him and ask him to come by for you?" In most cases, the patient is really just asking for someone to listen and that moment may pass by the time the chaplain visits. This means the chaplain should be training the nurses, home health aides, and others in how to react to spiritually oriented questions. The hospice must also provide resources—written and otherwise. One excellent written resource organizations may secure is the book *How to Be a Perfect Stranger: The Essential Religious Etiquette Handbook* by Stuart M. Matlins and Arthur Magida. There are many outside training avenues for the nurse and other team members such as the workshop provided by the Georgia Hospice Association in August 2010 on the subject of "Spiritual Care at the End of Life: Implementation, Integration and Inspiration."

In closing, it almost goes without saying that prior to hearing the spiritual needs of terminally ill patients, one must address the physical needs of the patient through effective pain management. It is difficult, although not impossible, to hear spiritual concerns through the physical agony and cries of those who are dying. Therefore, one of the most important things for a hospice organization to do in order to hear spiritual concerns is to deal effectively with pain. Then one can hear the primary concerns of the terminally ill patient, which were expressed so poignantly in the words of John Hardwig:

> When I am dying, I am quite sure that the central issues for me will not be whether I am put on a ventilator, whether CPR is administered when my heart stops, or whether I receive artificial feeding. Although each of these could be important, each will almost certainly be quite peripheral. Rather, my central concerns will be how to face death, how to bring my life to a close, and how best to help my family go on without me. (Hardwig, 2000, p. 28)

Dr. Richard B. Fife is a United Methodist minister, president of the Foundation for End-Of-Life Care in Ft. Lauderdale, Florida, and a founding and sustaining member of the Duke Institute for Care at the End of Life. A graduate of Duke University, Emory University, and Drew University, he was a parish minister for almost 20 years before becoming Vice President of Bioethics and Pastoral Care for VITAS Healthcare Corporation in Miami, Florida. He participated on the panel for the Hospice Foundation of America's 2005 Teleconference on ethics; and, among his writings are chapters on "Ethical Dilemmas in Hospice Care," "Diversity and Access to Hospice Care," and "Training for Diversity" in the Living with Grief *series by the Hospice Foundation of America.*

REFERENCES

Brenner, P. R. (2001). Spirituality in hospice. *The Park Ridge Center Bulletin, 21*, p. 3.

Byock, I., Norris, K., Strohmaier, G., & Asp, C. (2004, Jul–Aug). Spiritual care at the end of life. *Health Progress.*

Cobb, M. (2001). *The dying soul: Spiritual care at the end of life.* Buckingham, UK: Open University Press.

Doka, K., & Jenreski, M. (1985). Clergy understanding of grief, bereavement and mourning. *Research Record, 2*(4), 105–112.

Farleigh Hospice. (2008). *History of the hospice movement.* Available from http://www.farleigh.org

Frankl, V. (1963). *Man's search for meaning.* New York: Washington Square Press.

Hardwig, J. (2000). Spiritual issues at the end of life: A call for discussion. *Hastings Center Report, 30*(2), 28–30.

Howarth, G., & Leaman, O. (Eds.). (2001). Hospice in historical perspective. In *Encyclopedia of death and dying.* London: Routledge.

Matlins, S., & Magida, A. (1997). *How to be a perfect stranger: A guide to other people's religious ceremonies* (Vol. 2). Woodstock, VT: Jewish Lights Publishing.

Matlins, S., & Magida, A. (2010). *How to be a perfect stranger: The essential religious etiquette handbook* (5th ed.). Woodstock, VT: Skylight Paths Publishing.

National Hospice and Palliative Care Organization. (2009). *Guidelines for spiritual care in hospice.* Arlington, VA: National Hospice and Palliative Care Organization.

Saunders, C. (1960). Drug treatment in the terminal stages of cancer. *Current Medicine and Drugs 1*(1), 16–28.

Saunders, C. (1964, February 14). Care of patients suffering from terminal illness at St. Joseph's Hospice, Hackney, London. *Nursing Mirror,* vii–x.

Saunders, C. (1988). Spiritual pain. *Journal of Palliative Care, 4,* 29–32.

United States Code of Federal Regulation. (2009). Hospice Care, 42 C.F.R. pt. 418.

VITAS Healthcare Corporation, Suite 1500, 100 S. Biscayne Boulevard, Miami, Florida 33131.

Spiritual Perspectives on End-of-Life Care

This section reviews the perspectives of various religions on end-of-life care. When reviewing the data on religion, two things become clear. First, unlike Europeans, Americans are still generally a religious people. According to the American Religious Identification Survey (Kosmin & Keysar, 2008), over 80% of Americans still believe in a deity. Secondly, Americans are becoming more religiously diverse. While still overwhelmingly Christian with a smaller number of Jews, there is now a sustainable number of Muslims, Buddhists, and Hindus in the United States due to conversions and migrations from Africa, Asia, and the Middle East.

Somewhat less than 2% of Americans are Jewish. Kinzebrunner begins with a discussion of Jewish perspectives on end-of-life care. He offers a clear description of the beliefs and practices of Judaism and the ways these beliefs may influence care throughout the process of illness, dying, and grief. Kinzebrunner notes the differences between the varied perspectives within Judaism and shows special sensitivity to the needs and issues that may be experienced by holocaust survivors as they die.

A number of chapters describe the different varieties of Christianity, the faith of 76% of Americans (Kosmin & Keysar, 2008). Picci begins with Roman Catholics—around a quarter of all Americans. Picci describes the importance of the *Theology of the Cross*—the belief that in suffering, one shares in the suffering and redemption of Jesus—to the care of the dying. Picci also notes the importance placed on the sacraments and other rituals in Catholic practice. Harakas' chapter focuses on another branch of Christianity, Orthodoxy. Orthodox Christianity accounts for around 1% of Christians in the United States and has its roots in Greece, Russia, and Eastern Europe. Harakas especially notes the paradoxical Orthodox theology that in death, we are brought to eternal life. He then explores the mandates of that theology on end-of-life practices. Like Catholicism, sacrament and ritual play an important role in end-of-life care.

Protestants account for nearly two-thirds of American Christians. Nichols' chapter divides Protestantism into four distinct, yet not necessary mutually exclusive, categories: Mainline Protestantism, Evangelical/Fundamentalist Protestantism, Pentecostal/Charismatic Protestantism, and Anabaptist. Nichols' extensive review of these groups and the denominations within each group offer both helpful information and affirmation of the great diversity within the Protestant tradition. Sidebars here highlight three religious groups that arose in America: Jehovah's Witnesses, Christian Science, and the Church of Latter Day Saints (or Mormons), emphasizing particular practices that might influence end-of-life care.

Islam, while currently practiced by less than 1% of all Americans, is a rapidly growing faith in America. It is expected that sometime in the near future, Muslims might supplant Jews as the largest non-Christian faith in America. Hendi offers much here in his discussion of Islamic theology and practice at the end of life.

Hinduism and Buddhism, while still less than 1%, are also growing in the United States from both migrations and conversions. Kramer, in her chapter on Buddhism, asserts that the value of understanding Buddhist perspectives on death is twofold. First, Buddhism is one of the fastest growing religions in the United States. Hence, Kramer offers very practical guidelines for understanding ways to assist this emerging Buddhist population. Second, Kramer notes that Buddhism, with a strong belief in the impermanence of life and the truth of suffering, has much to contribute to compassionate care at the end of life. Chatterjee offers a rich chapter on Hinduism, noting how the call for conscious dying and certain burial practices may be sources of conflict with medical practice as well as economic and practical constraints.

Smith-Stoner's two chapters complete this section. The first chapter addresses those with less recognized spiritualities such as Wiccans, Pagans, and Nature Spiritualists, again around 1% of Americans. Her second chapter focuses on the growing numbers of agnostics, atheists, skeptics, humanists, and those who express little interest in any organized religion or theological orientation (or even oppose it)—now near 15% of the U.S. population. Smith-Stoner offers sound suggestions for sensitive practice, particularly to the hospice and palliative care communities whose very roots arise from the deep religious and spiritual orientation of its founder, Dame Cicely Saunders.

The chapters in this section make two additional points. One is that there is diversity within diversity; that is, there are considerable differences within a religion. This affirms a final point: an individual's spirituality should always be assessed. This closes the circle, reminding us once again that the shared religious beliefs of a faith community inform, but do not necessarily determine, the spirituality of its adherents.

REFERENCE

Kosmin, B., & Keysar, A. (2008). *American religious identification survey, 2008*. Hartford, CT: Trinity College.

CHAPTER 9

Jewish Perspectives on End-of-Life Care

Barry M. Kinzbrunner

Judaism, the most ancient of the monotheistic religions, traces its origins back to the Middle East well over 3,000 years ago. Fundamental to Jewish faith is the belief in one God, Who revealed Himself to Moses and the Jewish people on Mount Sinai. Jewish traditional belief and practice is embodied in Jewish law (known in Hebrew as *halacha*), which is derived primarily from the five books of Moses (the first five books of the Bible, known also to Jews as the *Torah*), the other books of the Jewish Bible, and an oral law that was later written down in the ancient texts of the *Mishnah* and *Talmud*, and subsequently expounded upon and codified by Jewish leaders throughout the last two millennia (Kinzbrunner, 2004; Lamm & Kinzbrunner, 2003).

There are approximately 5.5 million Jews in the United States today, representing a little over 1.5% of the total U.S. population. Approximately 10% of U.S. Jews identify themselves as Orthodox, meaning that they are observant of Jewish law and tradition and view the rabbi as the legal authority regarding Jewish law (Kinzbrunner, 2004). Conservative Jews, representing about 26% of the U.S. Jewish population, reinterpret Jewish law to fit modern society, exhibit wide variations in how they observe that reinterpreted law, and view the rabbi as an advisor rather than an authority figure (Dorff, 2003). Another 35% of Jews identify with Reform Judaism, which views Jewish law as only a nonbinding guide to living a moral and ethical life (Cutter, 2003). Another 9% of U.S. Jews are affiliated with several other small nontraditional denominations, and the remaining 20% are considered unaffiliated (Kotler-Berkowitz, Cohen, Ament, Klaff, Mott & Peckerman Neuman, 2004; Lamm & Kinzbrunner, 2003; Singer & Grossman, 2006).

From the information above, it would seem that most American Jews do not strictly observe Jewish law and tradition. While this assumption is generally correct, when the end of life approaches, many Jews, as people of other faiths, often look toward their beliefs and traditions as sources of aid and comfort during those difficult times. Hence, for both observant Jews and those who are less traditional, Jewish law and ritual can often significantly influence their wishes when they or members of their families become terminally ill.

END-OF-LIFE-CARE DECISION-MAKING

As the basis for healthcare decision-making under Jewish law, the cardinal ethical principles of medical ethics, autonomy, beneficence, nonmaleficence, and justice have been redefined from a Jewish perspective. Of the four, autonomy is most affected by this redefinition, for while Judaism believes in the concept of freedom of choice, a traditional Jew uses that freedom by choosing to follow God's law. Therefore, autonomy, defined in secular medical ethics as the right of an individual to choose among various care options (Kinzbrunner, 2002), is considered under its Jewish definition to be voluntarily limited from the perspective that a Jew will only consider those care options that are consistent with Jewish law (Steinberg, 1994, 2003).

The remaining values are more or less consistent with their secular medical ethical counterparts. Beneficence, the obligation to do what is good, is fully operational and in addition to the physician's ethical obligation to heal and provide beneficial care to patients, individuals have the obligation to care for themselves and seek beneficial care. Nonmaleficence, the avoidance of harm, is also incumbent on both the physician and the individual, within the constraints of an appropriate and acceptable risk/benefit analysis. Justice has both a societal component, the evaluation of the needs of the society as a whole, and a distributive component, which recognizes that there are finite resources to meet various healthcare needs (Steinberg, 1994, 2003).

Using these modified definitions of the ethical principles and other Jewish legal precepts, various decisions regarding care at the end of life can be made that are consistent with Jewish law, several of which will be discussed below, primarily from the traditional, Orthodox point of view. Hospice and palliative care professionals must recognize there may be significant differences of opinion on these issues among Jews who identify with the Conservative, Reform, or other non-Orthodox denominations, with the non-Orthodox tending to lean more toward a secular point of view (Dorff, 2003; Cutter, 2003). One must also be aware that even among traditional, Orthodox Jews and the rabbis who guide them, there are going to be differences of opinion on these various topics (Kinzbrunner, 2004). Therefore, when all is said and done, one must remember that when delivering culturally sensitive care, one can learn about how the group views a specific issue, but one must always look to each individual patient or patient-family unit to know how to provide proper care to best meet their specific needs.

Judaism teaches that life is of infinite value, so much so that the various restrictions in activities associated with observing the Sabbath are suspended when a life is at risk. Nevertheless, as King Solomon said in the Book of Ecclesiastes (3:2), Judaism recognizes that "there is a time live and a time to die." In keeping with that idea, traditional Judaism defines an individual as terminally ill if he or she has an illness that will prove fatal despite standard medical intervention within 1 year or less (Feinstein, 1996; Steinberg, 2003). A second type of terminally ill patient is called in Hebrew a *goses*, and this term is reserved for patients who would be described in hospice and palliative care as "actively dying" (Feinstein, 1996; Schostak, 2000).

Euthanasia, assisted suicide, or any other form of intentional hastening of death is categorically forbidden (Herring, 1984; Rosner, 2001). Patients who are near the end of life may refuse treatments that are deemed ineffective, futile, or will only prolong suffering, and such treatments may also be withheld. However, once treatments are started, they generally cannot be withdrawn, especially if they are considered to be life supportive in nature, since withdrawal of such treatment may be seen as an active shortening of life (Tendler & Rosner, 1996; Feinstein, 1996a).

Food and fluid, even when provided by artificial means, are considered by all Orthodox (Feinstein, 1996a; Berman, 1997; Schostak, 2000) and some Conservative rabbis (Reisner, 1990) to be basic care, and therefore, must be provided to all patients, with the only caveat being that this should be done in a way that is beneficial and not harmful. For other Conservative rabbis (Dorff, 1990), and rabbis of other non-Orthodox denominations (Dorff, 2003; Cutter, 2003), artificial hydration and nutrition are considered medical interventions and may be withheld or withdrawn based on the individual patient's, family's, or designated surrogate's wishes.

Advance directives in the form of a living will, a durable healthcare power of attorney, or both, are generally permitted and organizations from all the major Jewish denominations have advance directive documents that are compatible with their understanding and interpretation of Jewish law. An important requirement for advance directives in the Orthodox community, where the rabbi is the accepted authority on Jewish law, is that a rabbi knowledgeable in the area of healthcare decision-making must be included as a named surrogate in order to ensure that all such decisions are made in accordance with Jewish law (Lamm & Kinzbrunner, 2003; Kinzbrunner, 2004).

JEWISH TRADITIONS AND RITUALS

Prayer

Jews are obligated to pray three times every day. When possible, a minimum of 10 Jewish men (or either gender in non-Orthodox sects) gather together in synagogue for prayer in a group called a *minyan*, which is necessary for the recitation of certain prayers, including the mourner's *Kaddish* prayer. During weekday morning prayers, Jewish men (and some women in the Conservative movement) wear a prayer shawl, called a *tallit*, and *tefillin*, which are black leather boxes that are strapped onto the left upper arm and the forehead and contain parchment inscribed with specific scriptural verses. The tefillin are not worn during Sabbath or holiday prayers. The afternoon prayers are held late in the day followed by evening prayers, allowing Jews who attend daily services to only come to synagogue twice a day for the three prayer services (Lamm & Kinzbrunner, 2003).

Prayer may be a very important activity for patients and families during times of illness, even if the hope of recovery is very low. In addition to the thrice daily prayers, many Jews, whether observant or estranged from formal prayer, often find the recitation of Psalms (preferably using a direct Hebrew-English translation) to be a worthwhile and comforting activity. There are a large number of specific Psalms that are designated for this purpose (Scherman, 1990). There is also a formal prayer for the sick, referred to in Hebrew as the *Mi'sheberach*. While this is normally recited in synagogue following the reading of a portion from the Torah on Monday, Thursday, and Saturday mornings, caregivers may be asked by family members to recite this during a visit. Again, there are English translations available. At the point in the prayer when the name of the sick person is to be mentioned, it is customary to utilize the patient's Hebrew name, if known, and to identify the person as the son or daughter of his or her mother (rather than of the father, which is used in most other circumstances). When the individual is gravely ill, some have the custom of adding to or changing the sick person's name (Scherman, 1990).

Judaism has within its liturgy a confessional prayer, called *Vidui*, which is to be recited when one is about to die. A version of this prayer is recited as part of the prayers of repentance on specific occasions such as the Day of Atonement, Yom Kippur. While Jewish patients who are aware of the Vidui are often reluctant to recite it for fear it means they are definitely going to die, rabbis have always encouraged its recitation, reassuring the person by saying that not everyone who recites the prayer dies, and that its recitation ensures one a place in the "World to Come" (Karo, Shulchan Aruch, Yoreh Deah 338:1; Lamm & Kinzbrunner, 2003).

Sabbath and Holidays

Traditional Jews observe the Sabbath weekly on Saturday as a day of rest to commemorate the fact that following the six days of the creation of the world, God rested on the seventh day. During the Jewish Sabbath, which begins about one-half hour before sundown on Friday evening and ends one-half hour after sundown on Saturday night, Jews who follow the tradition are prohibited from performing many common weekday activities, including using electricity, cooking, carrying in a public domain, and traveling by a motor vehicle, to name but a few. There are many rituals associated with the Sabbath, including the lighting of candles, the sanctification of the day over wine, a family meal on Friday night, a longer synagogue service with the reading of a portion from the five Books of Moses from a handwritten parchment known as the Torah scroll, and another family meal, the Sabbath lunch.

There are also a number of Jewish holidays associated with many customs and rituals. Some of the better known Jewish holidays include Passover (during which Jews gather for a special meal called the *Seder* and eat unleavened bread called *matzah*), Rosh Hashanah (the Jewish New Year on which a ram's horn called a *shofar* is sounded), Yom Kippur (the Day of Atonement, a day of fasting and repentance), and Chanukah (the Festival of Lights during which Jews light a special candelabra for 8 nights). A number of the holidays, including Passover, Rosh Hashana, and Yom Kippur, have activity restrictions similar to the Jewish Sabbath (Lamm & Kinzbrunner, 2003).

While not all American Jews strictly observe the Sabbath or Jewish holidays in terms of ritual or activity restrictions, there are two important reasons why these special days on the Jewish calendar should become familiar to end-of-life caregivers caring for Jewish patients and families. Regarding the activity restrictions on the Sabbath and major Jewish holidays, all such restrictions are set aside when someone has a life-threatening illness, even if the person is terminal and not expected to recover (Kinzbrunner, 2004). Therefore, while end-of-life care providers should not meet any major challenges when caring for their patients and families on the Sabbath or a holiday, one should be aware that there will be situations where individual patients or family members who observe these restrictions may not be aware that the Sabbath and holiday prohibitions may be set aside, or may believe that the current medical situation is not severe enough to warrant violating the Sabbath or holiday. Therefore, it is important for caregivers to be aware of and sensitive to patient and family concerns when questions of Sabbath and holiday observance arise.

In regard to various rituals on the Sabbath and holidays, assisting patients in observing some of the rituals can be very meaningful, when due to the nature of their illnesses, they are unable to participate in the rituals on their own. Assisting an end-of-life care patient in lighting the Chanukah menorah, arranging for a rabbi to blow Shofar for a patient on Rosh Hashanah, or ensuring that a patient can light Shabbat candles are examples of how end-of-life caregivers can support Jewish patients and families who find these rituals important and meaningful (Lamm & Kinzbrunner, 2003).

Jewish Dietary Laws (Kosher)

The Jewish dietary laws (termed *Kosher*) are outlined in the Torah and elaborated upon by the rabbis in the oral law. These laws are followed by Orthodox Jews and, to varying degrees, by Jews affiliated with the Conservative and Reform movement. These laws include eating meat from only certain kinds of animals and birds that are slaughtered and then prepared in a specific fashion, eating only fish that have fins and scales, and not cooking or eating meat and dairy products together. Those who observe the Jewish dietary laws keep separate dishes for meat and dairy foods as well. Caregivers need to be aware of these restrictions and make sure they do not inadvertently bring nonkosher food into a patient's home (or kosher nursing home) or use the wrong dishes if they are assisting a patient or family member at mealtime. Caregivers should also be aware that even foods certified as kosher may not be considered acceptable to all Jews who state they follow the dietary laws and one should always check with the patient or family before bringing any foods into the home (Lamm & Kinzbrunner, 2003).

Modesty and Inter-Gender Contact

To varying degrees, Orthodox Jews refrain from any physical contact with members of the opposite gender with the exception of spouses and other immediate family members in the privacy of their own homes. Additionally, there may be concerns about patients of one gender being examined or otherwise cared for by a caregiver of the opposite gender in a secluded environment. While, like the laws of the Sabbath, these prohibitions are suspended when someone is ill, professional caregivers should be aware that some Orthodox patients may be extremely uncomfortable when care, especially personal care, is provided by a member of the opposite gender. Therefore, when an Orthodox Jewish patient requests that care be rendered by a caregiver of the same gender, it is incumbent upon end-of-life care providers to be respectful and flexible in order to meet the needs of such patients without subjecting them to undue stress (Weinreb, 2003; Steinberg, 2003; Kinzbrunner, 2009).

HOLOCAUST SURVIVORS

The specter of the systematic murder of the Jewish population of Europe by Nazi Germany during World War II, otherwise known as the holocaust, continues to cast its shadow over the last of its survivors, who are now dying of old age. Whether Jewish holocaust survivors observe Jewish law and ritual or not, their experiences during this period significantly color how they approach the natural end of their lives and greatly influences their end-of-life care decisions. For example, the mandate to provide artificial nutrition and hydration is not only due to basic human needs for these patients, but for many, reflects the overwhelming fear of starvation that was part and parcel of daily life under the Nazi yoke.

Challenges that end-of-life care providers may encounter when caring for elderly holocaust survivors may include exaggerated responses to pain and other symptoms (Barile, 2000) and a form of post-traumatic stress disorder, which, when coupled with the cognitive impairment that is common in the elderly, may cause them to become frightened by otherwise innocent stimuli such as hearing a dog bark, seeing a white lab coat, or being cared for by someone who speaks with a foreign accent (Goodman, 2003). Professional caregivers must be able to recognize these and other potentials problems that may be unique to the terminally ill holocaust survivor and be able to effectively manage any issues that arise.

THE AFTERLIFE IN JEWISH TRADITION

As belief or knowledge that life does not end with physical death may provide comfort and support to individuals who are dying, as well as those left behind to grieve, it is appropriate to briefly discuss how Jewish tradition views the afterlife. Life after death in Judaism may manifest itself in several ways. Following death, the soul will leave the body and continue to exist in the World of Souls, residing in *Gan Eden* (heaven) or, if necessary, first spending time in *Gehinnom* (a place of punishment, which is for a maximum of 12 months following which the soul goes to *Gan Eden*). Although generally thought of as a Christian concept, Judaism also believes in resurrection of the dead, with the world following resurrection sometimes referred to in Jewish literature as the "World to Come," although others use this term when referring to the World of Souls (Kaplan, 1993; Elias & Katz, 1995). Additionally, within the body of Jewish mysticism is the belief in reincarnation of the soul (Pinson, 1999).

As a caveat, it must be pointed out that Jews hold a wide variety of beliefs and opinions on the nature of life after death, based primarily on their level of religious observance and knowledge, ranging from belief in all the various manifestations of the afterlife to believing that there is no existence at all after death.

CARE OF THE BODY AT THE TIME OF DEATH

During the dying process, it is preferable that the patient not be left unattended. Once death occurs, it is customary for the children, close relatives, or friends who are present to close the deceased's eyes and draw a sheet over the face. The body is generally positioned so that the feet face the doorway, but is otherwise not moved. Candles are often lit, and there are various traditions as to how many and where. It is customary for friends and relatives to ask forgiveness of the deceased, and it is improper to eat or drink in the presence of the body (Lamm, 1969; Lamm & Kinzbrunner, 2003).

Cleaning and preparation of the body for internment is traditionally done by the *Chevra Kadisha*, the Jewish Burial Society, and includes the *taharah*, or ritual cleansing, and the recitation of specific prayers. Therefore, if a Jewish patient is having a traditional Jewish burial, end-of-life care staff should not clean the body at the time of death, but should leave the body and allow the Chevra Kadisha to remove all dressings, catheters, and other medical paraphernalia (Lamm & Kinzbrunner, 2003).

The deceased is dressed in a simple white shroud and a male (or in some Conservative and Reform groups both male and female) is then wrapped in his (or her) tallit (prayer shawl), with one set of the corner fringes (called *tzitzit*) cut off, making it unfit to be worn. The body is then placed in a coffin made entirely of wood, which decomposes at a rate similar to the body and the cloth. It is customary to drill holes in the bottom of the casket in order to connect the body more directly with the earth to which it will be returning (Lamm, 1969; Koltach, 1996; Lamm & Kinzbrunner, 2003).

From the time of death until the funeral, the body of the deceased is never left alone, but is attended to by a watcher (*shomer* in Hebrew) who recites various Psalms until the funeral. Autopsies are generally not permitted and if they are necessary, all organs must be returned for proper burial. Embalming and cremation are generally forbidden, although currently some groups within the Reform movement permit cremation (Koltach, 1996; Cutter, 2003).

THE FUNERAL AND INTERNMENT OF THE BODY

Burial usually occurs within 24 hours of death. The service includes various Psalms and prayers and a eulogy intended to praise the life of the deceased. Prior to the funeral, the primary mourners will perform *keriyah*, the tearing of a garment, as a demonstration of grief (Lamm, 1969). Conservative and reform Jews often choose to wear a torn black ribbon instead of tearing an article of clothing (Koltach, 1996; Cutter, 2003). Following the service, the mourners accompany the deceased to the gravesite and actually participate in the burial by shoveling earth into the grave until the coffin is entirely covered. Then, following the recitation of a special mourner's Kaddish prayer, the bereaved retire to the house of mourning, after being consoled by those who were present at the funeral and burial service (Lamm, 1969; Koltach, 1996; Lamm & Kinzbrunner, 2003).

The Kaddish Prayer

The Kaddish prayer is a central prayer in Jewish liturgy. It is recited in Aramaic, which was the common language of the people in ancient Israel and it can only be recited in the presence of a minyan. The theme of the prayer is praise of God, and there is no mention of death or mourning. It is recited multiple times during a traditional Jewish prayer service, often serving to separate various parts of the daily service from one another. It is also recited following the reading of certain Jewish texts of learning, and, in the context of mourning and bereavement, is recited by someone who is in mourning.

Because of its familiarity to most Jews, the recitation of Kaddish during periods of mourning can quickly become rote and automatic for many. As that occurs, and the mind of the mourner reciting the prayer begins to wander, it allows the individual to think about and even communicate in some way with the deceased, allowing the bereaved to better cope with his loss (Lamm, 1969; Lamm & Kinzbrunner, 2003; Lamm, 2004).

MOURNING AND BEREAVEMENT CUSTOMS

There are seven relatives whose loss obligates a Jewish adult (male over the age of 13, female over the age of 12) to mourn: father, mother, sister, brother, son, daughter, and spouse. Traditional Jewish practice defines four stages of mourning: *aninus*, *shiva*, *sheloshim*, and a final period that is only observed following the death of a parent, which ends 12 months after the loss.

Aninus

The first stage of mourning is called aninus and it encompasses the period between the death and burial of the loved one. Despair is usually very intense (even when death is expected), yet, at the same time, the bereaved is expected to focus on ensuring that all final arrangements for the deceased have been made. In recognition of this, in addition to refraining from the social and personal activities that are traditionally forbidden during mourning, the mourner is not obligated to participate in certain religious observances related to prayer (Lamm, 1969; Lamm & Kinzbrunner, 2003).

Shiva

Shiva begins following the funeral and traditionally lasts for 7 days, although some Conservative and Reform Jews choose to only observe 3 days or 1 day (Koltach, 1996; Cutter, 2003). During the first 3 days of the traditional shiva period, mourning is particularly intense, and the mourner does not traditionally respond to greetings. During the final 4 days, the mourner begins to emerge from the state of intense grief and is more prepared to talk about the loss (Lamm, 1969; Lamm & Kinzbrunner, 2003).

During the shiva period, mourners will traditionally wear the garment or black ribbon that was torn or cut during the funeral, will sit on a low stool, and will wear slippers. Mourners are also restricted in a number of activities. They are not permitted to leave the house, shave and groom, bathe for pleasure, work or conduct normal business activities, wear new or freshly laundered clothes, and engage in conjugal relations. It is traditional for friends to visit mourners during the shiva period to express condolences and provide emotional support. A candle is lit that will last the entire 7-day shiva period, and all the mirrors in the home are covered (Lamm, 1969; Lamm & Kinzbrunner, 2003).

The traditional obligations for daily prayer that were suspended during aninus are resumed following the funeral, with the addition of the mourner's Kaddish prayer. As the mourners traditionally do not leave the house, it is common in traditional Jewish communities to conduct prayer services in the house of mourning (Lamm, 1969; Koltach, 1996; Lamm & Kinzbrunner, 2003).

Sheloshim

This stage of mourning represents the 30 days following burial, and includes the 7 days of shiva. After shiva, the mourner is encouraged to leave the house and begin to reintegrate into society. Certain activities, such as shaving and grooming, and attending parties and other celebratory functions with music remain prohibited under normal circumstances during the sheloshim period. Recitation of the Kaddish remains an obligation of the mourners during sheloshim. However, rather than holding services for the bereaved in the home, they can attend services in the community synagogue. Sheloshim concludes mourning obligations for the loss of all relatives except for one's parents (Lamm, 1969; Lamm & Kinzbrunner, 2003).

Final Mourning Period of 12 Months for One's Parent

Due to the special relationship that a child has to his or her parents, the loss of a parent is more keenly felt. Therefore, an extra period of mourning is proscribed. While business and many other activities return to normal, entertainment and amusement activities are curtailed for a period of 12 months following the funeral. Recitation of Kaddish during daily prayers also continues until the end of the 11th month (Lamm, 1969; Koltach, 1996; Lamm & Kinzbrunner, 2003).

MEMORIALIZING THE DECEASED AFTER FORMAL BEREAVEMENT

While organized bereavement is discontinued after 1 year (or 30 days for other relatives), Jewish tradition continues to encourage the remembrance of those who have passed on. Toward the end of the year of mourning for a parent (or following the sheloshim for other relatives), it is not uncommon for the bereaved to gather at the gravesite of the deceased to unveil the headstone of the grave. This custom, called an "Unveiling," has its origins in 19th century America and Western Europe and, in addition to the unveiling of the headstone, includes the recitation of some Psalms, a brief eulogy, the special memorial prayer recited at the funeral, and the Kaddish prayer. This affords the mourners another opportunity to remember the deceased (Lamm, 1969; Koltach, 1996).

On the yearly anniversary of the death of a loved one, or *Yahrzeit*, Kaddish is recited during prayer in remembrance of the deceased and a memorial candle is lit. Judaism also has special prayers of remembrance, the *Yizkor* service, which are recited 4 times a year, during the three major festivals (Passover, Shavuot, and Succot) and on Yom Kippur, to honor all those who have passed on (Lamm, 1969; Koltach, 1996).

When reflecting on the stages of mourning discussed above, one can see that this represents a model of healthy bereavement activities. The bereaved appropriately experience intense grieving at the time of the loss, followed by a structured decrease in the grief process, with a concomitant normalization of day-to-day activities (Lamm, 1969; Lamm & Kinzbrunner, 2003; Lamm, 2004).

Rabbi Barry M. Kinzbrunner, MD, FACP, FAAHPM, is executive vice-president and chief medical officer for VITAS Healthcare Corporation in Miami, Florida. He is board certified in internal medicine, medical oncology, and hospice and palliative medicine and he was ordained as an Orthodox rabbi in Jerusalem, Israel, in 2002. During his more than 25-year career in hospice and palliative medicine, Rabbi Dr. Kinzbrunner has spoken and published extensively on the care of patients at the end of life, including a textbook titled 20 Common Problems in End-of-Life Care, *for which a second edition under the new title* End of Life Care: A Practical Guide *was released at the end of 2010. Rabbi Dr. Kinzbrunner has also developed expertise in end-of-life care issues pertaining to patients of the Jewish faith and has published and lectured extensively in this area. Since 1998, he has been consulting with JDC-Eshel in Israel to help develop hospice and palliative care services in Israel, including the development of spiritual care services in Israel in cooperation with the National Association of Jewish Chaplains. He has been married since 1974, and is the father of three sons, ages 30, 27, and 22.*

REFERENCES

Barile, A. (2000, March–April). Geriatric study of survivors. *International Society for Yad Vashem, Martyrdom and Resistance, 14.*

Berman, A. (1997). From the legacy of Rav Moshe Feinstein. *Journal of Halacha and Contemporary Society, 13,* 5–18.

Cutter, W. (2003). Reform Judaism & secular Jewish practice. In M. Lamm & B. M. Kinzbrunner (Eds.), *The Jewish hospice manual: A guide to compassionate end-of-life care for Jewish patients and their families.* Miami, FL: VITAS Healthcare Corporation and National Institute for Jewish Hospice.

Dorff, E. N. (1990). A Jewish approach to end-stage medical care. *Proceedings of the Committee on Jewish Law and Standards, 1986–1990*. Retrieved January 20, 2006 from http://www.rabbinicalassembly.org/teshuvot/docs/19861990/dorff_care.pdf

Dorff, E. N. (2003). Conservative & reconstructionist Judaism. In M. Lamm & B. M. Kinzbrunner (Eds.), *The Jewish hospice manual: A guide to compassionate end-of-life care for Jewish patients and their families*. Miami, FL: VITAS Healthcare Corporation and National Institute for Jewish Hospice.

Elias, J., & Katz, D. (1995). The messianic era, the resurrection of the dead, and the world to come. In *The Art Scroll Series, Schottenstein Edition, Talmud Bavli, Tractate Sanhedrin* (vol. 3.) (Appendix). Brooklyn, NY:, Mesorah Publications.

Feinstein, M. (1996). Iggeros Moshe, Choshen Mishpat II: 73. In M. D. Tendler, *Responsa of Rav Moshe Feinstein, v. 1, care of the critically ill* (pp. 38–53). Hoboken, NJ: Ktav Publishing House.

Feinstein, M. (1996a). Iggeros Moshe, Choshen Mishpat II: 74. In M. D. Tendler, *Responsa of Rav Moshe Feinstein, v. 1, care of the critically ill* (pp. 53–62). Hoboken, NJ: Ktav Publishing House.

Goodman, R. (2003). Aging survivors with cognitive loss. In P. David & S. Pelly (Eds.), *Caring for aging holocaust survivors: A practice manual*. Toronto: Baycrest Centre for Geriatric Care.

Herring, B. F. (1984). Euthanasia. In B.F. Herring, *Jewish ethics and halakha for our time, sources and commentary, v. 1* (pp 67–90). New York: Ktav Publishing House.

Kaplan, A. (1993). On the resurrection. In A. Kaplan, *Immortality, resurrection, and the age of the universe: A Kabbalistic view* (pp. 29–44). Hoboken, NJ: Ktav Publishing House.

Karo, J. *Shulchan Aruch Yoreh Deah*, 338:1.

Kinzbrunner, B. M. (2002). Introduction. In B. M. Kinzbrunner, N. J. Weinreb & J. Policzer (Eds.), *Twenty common problems in end-of-life care* (pp *xi–xiv*). New York: McGraw Hill.

Kinzbrunner, B. M. (2004). Jewish medical ethics and end-of-life care. *Journal of Palliative Medicine, 7*(4), 558–573.

Kinzbrunner, B. M. (2009). Orthodox and Hasidic perspectives. In K. J. Doka & A. S. Tucci (Eds.), *Living with grief: Diversity and end-of-life care* (pp. 142–150). Washington, DC: Hospice Foundation of America.

Koltach, A. J. (1996). *The Jewish mourner's book of why.* Middle Village: Jonathan David Publishers.

Kotler-Berkowitz, L., Cohen, S. M., Ament, J., Klaff, V., Mott, F., & Peckerman-Neuman, D. (2004). *National Jewish population survey, 2000–2001: Strength, challenge, and diversity in the American Jewish population.* New York: United Jewish Communities.

Lamm, M. (1969). *The Jewish way in death and mourning.* New York: Jonathan David Publishers.

Lamm, M. (2004). *Consolation: The spritual journey beyond grief.* Philadelphia, PA: Jewish Publication Society.

Lamm, M., & Kinzbrunner, B. M. (2003). *The Jewish hospice manual: A guide to compassionate end-of-life care for Jewish patients and their families.* Miami, FL: VITAS Healthcare Corporation and National Institute for Jewish Hospice.

Pinson, D. (1999). *Reincarnation and Judaism.* Northvale, NJ: Jason Aronson, Inc.

Reisner, A. I. (1990). A Halachic ethic of care for the terminally ill. Proceedings of the *Committee on Jewish Law and Standards, 1986-1990.* Retrieved January 20, 2006 from http://www.rabbinicalassembly.org/teshuvot/docs/19861990/reisner_care.pdf

Rosner, F. (2001). Euthanasia. In F. Rosner (Ed.), *Biomedical ethics and Jewish law* (pp. 271–285). Hoboken, NJ: Ktav Publishing House.

Scherman, N. (1990). *The complete art scroll siddur. A new translation and anthologized commentary* (3rd ed.), (pp. 1040–1041). Brooklyn, NJ: Mesorah Publications.

Schostak, Z. (2000). Precedents for hospice and surrogate decision-making in Jewish law. *Tradition, 34*(2), 40–57.

Singer, D., & Grossman, L. (Eds.) (2006). *American Jewish yearbook, 2006.* New York: American Jewish Committee. Retrieved October 15, 2008 from http://www.jewishvirtuallibrary.org/jsource/US-Israel/usjewpop.html

Steinberg, A. (1994). A Jewish perspective on the four principles. In R. Gillon & A. Lloyd (Eds.), *Principles of healthcare ethics* (pp. 65–73). Chichester, England: John Wiley and Sons.

Steinberg, A. (2003). Encyclopedia of Jewish medical ethics (F. Rosner, Trans.) Jerusalem: Feldheim Publications.

Tendler, M. D., & Rosner, F. (1996). Quality and sanctity of life in the Talmud and Midrash. In M. D. Tendler, *Responsa of Rav Moshe Feinstein, v. 1, care of the critically ill* (pp. 135–148). Hoboken, NJ: Ktav Publishing House.

Weinreb, T. H. (2003). Hasidic and ultra-orthodox Judaism. In M. Lamm & B. M. Kinzbrunner (Eds.), *The Jewish hospice manual: A guide to compassionate end-of-life care for Jewish patients and their families.* Miami, FL: VITAS Healthcare Corporation and National Institute for Jewish Hospice.

CHAPTER 10

Discovering the Sacrament of the Present Moment: Catholic Spiritual Practices at the End of Life

Tina Picchi

I remember how my heart ached with sadness as I entered the nursing home where my father lived. I experienced such heavy-heartedness and a sense of loss as I searched for him among the frail elderly residents. At times I could barely recognize my father as he looked so disheveled and estranged from himself.

My father, Ambrose, spent his last 8 years in dementia care institutions. He lost his memory, ability to speak, and his independence. A certified public accountant with a distinguished career in the Internal Revenue Service, he could no longer comprehend the value of currency. For the most part, he did not recognize his family. Painfully, his illness robbed him of most things that brought him pleasure, with one exception. He did not lose his enjoyment of fine food. Consequently, my visits to him usually included a trip to an Italian deli to buy him a gourmet sandwich or the pasta of the day and of course, dessert. Our time together was focused on this meal, a welcome change from the daily hospital fare. He had a look of complete contentment as he enjoyed bites of these delicacies.

I treasure the memory of these midday feasts that transformed our visits and became a shared communion between father and daughter. For a brief period, it was as if time was suspended, his memory was restored, and he was able to recognize me as family once again. Since his death, I have come to realize that this transformation was mutual. In offering him familiar foods and experiencing his delight, the veil was lifted from my eyes and I was able to appreciate my father for who he had become. He was not lost to me. We were present to each other in a new way. This presence was sheer gift that took us to a place beyond words where spirits meet and souls embrace.

These encounters with my father remind me of a Biblical story from the Gospel of Luke where Jesus' disciples were walking down the road from Jerusalem to a town named Emmaus a few days after Jesus had been crucified. Their hearts were heavy with a profound sense of loss. Jesus appears to the disciples on their journey but in their sorrow they are unable to recognize him. Only when they stop along the road to share a meal with this stranger are their eyes opened and they recognize him in the breaking of the bread. The disciples were amazed that they were with Jesus all day and only recognized him for a brief moment before he once again vanished from their sight (Luke 24: 13–35).

In my early years of studying Catholic theology, I discovered Jean-Pierre de Caussade's extraordinary spiritual work, *Abandonment to Divine Providence*. This classic spiritual text has guided me in my spiritual journey and pastoral ministry ever since. Jean-Pierre was an early 18th century French Jesuit priest, theologian, and spiritual director. He emphasizes the importance of embracing "the sacrament of the present moment" (de Caussade, 1975, p. 24) and reminds his readers that although the activity of God may be invisible to us in times of suffering and indignity, if we are patient and practice vigilant attention, the veil will be lifted and we will be surprised and rejoice in God's active presence in our lives. "If we live by faith we shall judge things very differently from the way people who rely on their senses and so remain unaware of the priceless treasure hidden under appearances" (p. 38).

Discovering the Spirit of Another

In my role as a Catholic hospital chaplain, I adopted a simple definition for spiritual care that I believe describes the essence of responding to spiritual needs. Spiritual care is discovering, reverencing, and tending the spirit of another. Discovering who a person is and what they hold sacred is a tremendous gift. We learn what really matters to an individual and what is vital to their wholeness. There is always an element of mystery when we encounter another person. It is essential that we approach him or her with deep reverence and respect for the individual's beliefs and core values. If we are invited into the inner landscape of their soul, it is a privilege and a trust that we must never take for granted. Discovering the spirit of another requires deep presence and intent listening to both words and nonverbal expressions. We pay attention to the "sacrament of the present moment." As spiritual care providers, we help others uncover and embrace what brings beauty, hope, peace, courage, and a sense of right relationship and deeper connection with the significant and sacred into their lives.

In the introductory story about my father, I offered a glimpse into the experience of being present to him after he had lost the capacity to communicate meaningfully through words and concepts. I discovered that it was above all else, sharing a special meal that served as a bridge to a deeper awareness of each other and a reverencing of the moments shared. This was very satisfying for me both as a daughter and a chaplain. Because of his profound dementia, he was no longer able to attend Mass or receive communion. These religious practices had been very important to him as a Catholic all of his life. Even so, I believe our encounters had a sacramental quality, as these shared meals were times of significant intimacy, lifting the veil from our eyes and revealing the presence of God in our midst. I gained new insight into why the celebration of Eucharist is such a central part of the Catholic faith. We hunger for bread that nourishes our bodies and nurtures our souls. We long to sit at table and belong to a family where there is true communion. We yearn to know that God understands our pain and suffering and desires to share intimately in our lives.

The experience of my father's final years was a valuable pastoral lesson in discovering what is significant, relevant, and possible for the patient and family at this point in their lives together and then responding with attentiveness and compassion. This is the starting point of spiritual care for the sick and those approaching the end of life. It is in this context of discovering, reverencing, and tending each individual's spiritual needs that I offer a perspective on spiritual beliefs and practices that are important to many Catholics, particularly at the end of life. I begin with the relevance of the sacraments.

SACRAMENTS

In the Catholic Church, there are seven sacraments that mark significant times of passage in our lives. These sacraments—celebrated in community—reveal the living and loving presence of God in the human experience and serve as transformational encounters. These sacred rituals are "moments of reflection, shared with one another in celebration that bring together and deepen all our other reflections about life. They are key experiences that provide new insights into our other experiences and deepen them" (Cooke, 1983, p. 12). The three sacraments most frequently celebrated at times of illness and impending death are Eucharist, the Sacrament of the Sick, and the Sacrament of Reconciliation.

Eucharist

Eucharist, as already mentioned, is central to the sacramental life of Catholics. During Mass, bread and wine are transformed into the body and blood of Christ and Catholics unite themselves in Christ's suffering, death, and resurrection. In the breaking of the bread and the sharing of the cup, the faith community is nourished and strengthened in their living and in their dying. As is true with all Catholic sacraments, Eucharist is celebrated in the context of community in recognition that those who gather around the table are the Body of Christ, united in the solemn act of worship with the whole communion of saints, both living and dead.

When members are unable to participate in the liturgy due to illness, disability, or advanced age, the Church provides Eucharistic ministry to the home-bound and institutionalized, a significant pastoral outreach. The priest, deacon, or lay Eucharistic minister provides this sacramental ministry in the context of a ritual that includes prayer and scripture and serves as a vital connection with the larger faith community. Eucharist as viaticum—food for the journey—is offered to Catholic patients who are dying, a strong reminder that God calls each person to share in the banquet of eternal life. Whenever possible, viaticum should be offered to persons in the early stages of dying when they are still conscious and able to receive communion in the presence of loved ones who are there to pray with them and help sustain them on their final journey (National Conference of Catholic Bishops, 1983, p. 45).

Anointing of the Sick
The sacrament of the Anointing of the Sick, scripturally rooted in the New Testament, calls upon the faith community to be present to the sick and dying in prayerful support and not abandon them at a time of great vulnerability.

> If one of you is ill, he should send for the elders of the church, and they must anoint him with oil in the name of the Lord and pray over him. The prayer of faith will save the sick man and the Lord will raise him up again; and if he has committed any sins, he will be forgiven. (James 5:14–15, The Jerusalem Bible)

Pain can overwhelm an individual's sense of being in control, instill fear, and intensify a sense of isolation and loneliness that contributes to intense suffering. Suffering affects not only the person's concept of self but their whole sense of connection to others and the world. The sacrament of the Anointing of the Sick seeks to restore the sick person's relationship within the community, relieve suffering, and sustain hope. This sacrament may be offered to any Catholic who is seriously ill or of advanced age and may be received at various times throughout an extended illness. It contains many healing elements: the blessing of the sick and those who care for them with holy water, a penitential rite for the forgiveness of sin, scripture readings that offer guidance and consolation, the laying on of hands, and the anointing of the sick person with blessed oil. A litany of prayers calls upon the saints and angels to guide and protect the sick and those who care for them.

In his final days, my father was unable to receive viaticum, the special Rite of Communion for those who are dying. We called for the priest to offer a final blessing in preparation for his death and were deeply touched by his humanity and kindness when he arrived at the nursing home. He understood the art of pastoral presence and how it served as a bridge to the sacramental encounter. He asked about our father's life and was engaged and attentive. He anointed my father with holy oils, extending a blessing upon him on behalf of the whole faith community and in particular, each of his seven children. It was a simple but beautiful ritual, very loving and filled with hope for the journey ahead.

Reconciliation

For many, dying is a time to attend to unfinished business and seek amends. The need for reconciliation, the restoration of right relationships with oneself, others, and God, is made even more acute in the face of death. Seeking and offering forgiveness has a profound impact on a patient and family preparing for death. Reconciliation brings a freedom of spirit and a peacefulness that helps both patient and family surrender to the inevitability of death. Expressing one's sorrow and seeking forgiveness in the sacrament of Reconciliation offers Catholics a pastoral opportunity to confess their sins and receive absolution from the priest. This sacrament offers deep spiritual healing and forgiveness and should be made available to any Catholic who requests it.

REVERENCING THE SPIRIT OF ANOTHER

> There is a season for everything, a time for every occupation under heaven:
> A time for giving birth, a time for dying;
> A time for planting, a time for uprooting what has been planted.
> A time for killing, a time for healing;
> A time for knocking down, a time for building;
> A time for tears, a time for laughter;
> A time for mourning, a time for dancing.
>
> (Ecclesiastes 3:1–4, TJB)

Each moment is pregnant with possibility. It is imperative to know precisely what time it is in one's life in order to recognize what work is yet to be done. For those living with chronic and life-limiting illness, it is essential that they receive the very best medical information possible about their disease process and its impact on the course and quality of their life. Ultimately, each individual must examine the benefits and burdens of treatment options in light of their own spirituality and what gives meaning and purpose to their living and their dying. Hospital chaplains play a vital role in helping individuals and families access information, articulate goals of care, and make choices about medical treatment that are consistent with the patient's own faith, beliefs, and values.

Awareness of death can profoundly raise an individual's consciousness of God, faith, and the meaning and purpose of one's life. Accepting the limits of one's life span can lead to a deeper appreciation for the gift of life and the importance of treasured relationships and honored commitments. Reconciliation with family, community, self, and God may become a priority. There is an urgency to use time well, to seek a sense of wholeness and completeness in one's life story. Death is the ultimate and inevitable spiritual experience. For Catholics, it is a journey of faith, strengthened by the belief that death is not an absolute end, but rather a transition from this life to the next where we will live in the presence of a loving and forgiving God, reunited with loved ones and the whole Communion of Saints.

TENDING THE SPIRIT OF ANOTHER

In *Beauty: The Invisible Embrace*, the Irish Catholic poet, theologian, and spiritual director John O'Donohue masterfully describes the holiness of dying and the importance of supporting and attending to the dying individual who is setting out on a solitary journey.

> A deathbed is such a special and sacred place; a deathbed is more like an altar than a bed. It is an altar where the flesh and blood of a life is transformed into eternal spirit. Rather than being unsure, anxious and bungling, we should endeavor to be present there with the most contemplative, priestly grace. Regardless of the shock and pain of our grief, our whole attention should be dedicated to the one who is setting off on their solitary journey. Now we need to provide the best shelter, the sweetest love, the most sensitive listening and the most wholesome words for the one who is dying. This is the most

> significant time, the last moments of time on earth. Therefore
> it is vital to attend and listen. Perhaps there are last things a
> person wishes to say, things from long-forgotten past times and
> always wished to say but never could. Before the great silence
> falls, he or she might desperately need to tell something. And
> there may be things that need to be heard. Perhaps someone
> around that deathbed has waited all their life to hear something,
> vitally healing and encouraging and perhaps these are the hours
> it might be heard. (O'Donohue, 2004, pp. 202–203)

When we tend to another at the end of life, we participate in a transformational journey as the dying person prepares to finish their life here on earth. It is our role to offer "the best shelter, the sweetest love, the most sensitive listening and the most wholesome words." We honor the sacredness of this time by creating a sanctuary where the individual can engage in the holy work of dying supported and accompanied by family and caregivers who respect the significance of the work that is being accomplished. Providing the "best shelter" for the dying also means letting others into our hearts and having the spiritual capacity to be truly open to another's pain and suffering. Standing with others at the crossroads of life and death requires courageous presence. This is symbolized in the Christian scriptures, when Mary and the other women remain faithfully present to Jesus on the cross as he is dying, even as others have fled in fear. To be courageously present to a suffering person is to enter into their vulnerability and risk becoming vulnerable ourselves. "To be vulnerable means there is a substantial risk that one's intrinsic dignity is not affirmed and one's worth or value as a member of the human community is not recognized" (Sulmasy, 2006, p. 33).

> The task of the healthcare professional is to show respect and
> reverence for the dignity all dying persons have simply because
> they are human; to share their own hope that meaning transcends
> the dying process; and to point the way to reconciliation. They can
> do nothing more. They must do nothing less. (Sulmasy, p. 209)

Within Catholic health care, there is a strong belief that attending to the dying is a hallmark of the Church's healing mission and there is a clear mandate to respect the dignity of each person by providing excellent physical, psychosocial, and spiritual care. This commitment to attend to the whole person is inspired by the vision of the early founders of religious communities who opened the first hospitals and is rooted in the Gospel where Jesus modeled a compassionate and healing response to many who suffered in body, mind, and spirit. Palliative care programs have become integral to Catholic health care as they seek to improve the quality of life for persons living with chronic and life-limiting illness and to ease the way for those who are dying. Palliative care recognizes that dying is not simply a biological event we witness but a sacred act that we are privileged to participate in. "The closer one comes to the edges of life, the more clearly one comes to confront the transcendent." (Sulmasy, p. 188)

SHARING IN THE CROSS AND SUFFERING OF JESUS

The call to share in Jesus' cross and redemptive suffering is a core belief for Catholics. In *The Gift of Peace* (1997), Cardinal Joseph Bernardin reflects on the meaning of his own suffering and death as he faces a diagnosis of terminal cancer. In his lovely meditation, *Suffering in Communion with the Lord*, he reflects on the essential mystery of the cross. Embracing one's cross, in communion with Jesus, gives rise to a certain kind of loneliness, an inability to see clearly how things are unfolding, an inability to see that, ultimately, all things will work for our good, and that we are, indeed, not alone. Participating in the paschal mystery of Jesus brings a certain freedom: the freedom to let go, to surrender ourselves to the living God and to place ourselves completely in God's hands. It is in the act of abandonment that we experience redemption and find life, peace, and joy in the midst of physical, emotional, and spiritual suffering. According to Bernardin, Christians must let the mystery, the tranquility, and the purposefulness of Jesus' suffering become part of their life before they can become effective instruments of God's healing for others (Bernardin, 1997, pp. 45–49).

THE WAY OF THE CROSS

Susan Catherine Mitchell, a Catholic hospice chaplain, authored an inspiring book titled *Through the Valley: The Way of the Cross for the End of Life* (2009) that serves as a spiritual pilgrimage for those facing serious illness and loss. In her preface she writes:

> The end of life is a deeply holy and intense time. It can be a time for growth, for connection among people and connection to the Divine. It can also be painful, sad, exhausting and draining, all at the same time. It is in this very intensity that we can break

through to an awareness of the God who sustains us, a God who is both the very fiber of our being and so transcendent that we are stopped wordless in wonder. We do not come to God apart from our daily lives, but through them. What has given meaning and purpose to us throughout our lives is what will give meaning and purpose to us during our final days. (Mitchell, 2009, p. 8)

The way of the cross is pictorially displayed in most Catholic Churches and referred to as the "Stations of the Cross." These stations are places of contemplation for Catholics to pause and reflect upon the meaning of Jesus' suffering, death, and resurrection in their own lives. They are an invitation for Christians to walk the path that Jesus walked and immerse themselves in the story of Jesus' journey of faith as he embraced his redemptive suffering and death on the cross.

OTHER SPIRITUAL PRACTICES AT THE END OF LIFE

For some Catholics, praying the rosary at the bedside of a dying family member is a very important communal ritual. The joyful, sorrowful, glorious, and luminous mysteries of the rosary are a scriptural meditation and guide to contemplating Mary and Jesus' faith and trust in God and include a repetition of prayers and intercessions to Mary. This traditional prayer has particular significance for some cultural groups and is prayed at the bedside of the dying and on subsequent days and anniversaries following the death.

Prayers of commendation for the dying, which include viaticum (communion service) whenever possible, offer scriptural reflections, litanies, and blessings for the person who is dying and for those who attend to them. These prayers can be offered by ordained members of the Church as well as lay Eucharistic ministers.

There are many Catholics who for one reason or another will not choose to receive sacraments or engage in other traditional Catholic rituals as they approach the end of life. As with any patient, it is important to explore what gives meaning and purpose to their life and what spiritual practices may offer them peace and hope. The reading from Ecclesiastes 3:1–8 can be an invitation to reflect upon the question "What is it time for?" and help the patient and family discover what sacred work needs to be done to bring life's relationships to completeness. Exploring themes of love, forgiveness, gratitude, leaving behind a legacy, and saying goodbyes can encourage individuals and families to engage in very personal and meaningful rituals that bring healing and wholeness. In some Catholic hospitals, music thanatologists create a peaceful, restful environment for the dying and music therapists offer music that facilitates the sharing of significant memories. Hospital volunteers provide lovely handmade prayer shawls or comfort quilts that are bestowed on the dying with blessings for the journey. Healing gardens are a place of respite for the sick and their family to spend time in the beauty of nature. Often family are invited to memorial ceremonies to honor loved ones who have died.

FUNERAL LITURGY

Asking individuals in advance how they would like to be remembered opens up important conversations within families and lessens the burden of decision-making regarding funeral arrangements. Too often families wait until after their loved one has died to begin planning the funeral, only to discover they are exhausted, overwhelmed, and have little time to create a service that truly honors the individuality of the deceased. Many Catholic parishes have bereavement and liturgy coordinators who can guide families in planning services that are personal and meaningful to loved ones and liturgically acceptable.

My father's funeral Mass was a return to the parish where we grew up, bringing together family, friends, and parishioners, many of whom we had known since childhood. It was followed by a family reunion at a local Italian restaurant. These arrangements were part of my father's careful planning from years earlier.

The theme of his funeral liturgy was "Come to the Table," celebrating how much he loved hosting big family meals. We envisioned him sitting at a huge banquet table in heaven, reunited with our mother, his parents and siblings, and the whole communion of saints, toasting to the occasion and enjoying his favorite foods. The first scripture described the heavenly banquet as a feast of rich food and choice wines (Isaiah 25:6). The priest who presided at the funeral Mass was a true pastor who was both inspiring and comforting. Though he had never met my father, he had taken careful note of the stories we had shared. During his homily, he had a special message for the grandchildren, many of whom barely remembered their grandfather before his long illness. He encouraged them to practice little acts of kindness to honor their grandfather's memory. This made a big impression on both the children and adults present.

My father's final years were both painful and profound. He did not "go gently into that good night" and before he lost his ability to speak, he cursed and "raged against the dying of the light" (Thomas, 2003, p. 122). As his illness progressed, I believe it was our shared Catholic faith and traditions that encompassed us like a mighty fortress and gave us both the courage and stamina to endure the mystery of this suffering. Scripture and sacrament illuminated the darkness of this very difficult experience. There were moments of transformation, when the veil was lifted and through the eyes of faith, I was able to know my father and be known. These experiences were ones of surprise and delight when I was able to discover the hidden activity of God, in the sacrament of the present moment. These breakthrough moments were sheer gift! In many ways my father was my teacher. I learned the importance of practicing patience and vigilance in discovering reverencing and tending the spirit of another. I believe there is always an opening, no matter how small, that allows us to truly encounter another person and come to know them in ways beyond words and concepts, a place where spirits meet and souls embrace.

Tina Picchi, currently living in Portland, Oregon, is executive director of the Supportive Care Coalition, a national collaborative of 19 Catholic healthcare organizations dedicated to pursuing excellence in palliative care through knowledge transfer, advocacy, and partnerships. A Catholic chaplain and board-certified by the National Association of Catholic Chaplains for over 30 years, Ms. Picchi holds a bachelor of arts in theology from the University of San Francisco and a master of arts in applied spiritual theology from Mount St. Mary's College in Los Angeles. She has extensive healthcare leadership experience in spiritual care, ethics, and mission integration, as well as palliative care. Most recently, she directed palliative care services for two Catholic hospitals in Southern California where she initiated and developed a nationally recognized palliative care program with an innovative transdisciplinary team of health professionals.

REFERENCES

Bernardin, J. (1997). *The gift of peace: Personal reflections.* Chicago: Loyola.

Cooke, B. (1983). *Sacraments and sacramentality.* Mystic, CT: Twenty-Third Publication.

de Caussade, P. (1975). *Abandonment to divine providence.* (J. Beavers, Trans.). Garden City, NY: Image Books.

Jones, A. (Ed.). (1966). *The Jerusalem Bible.* Garden City, NY: Doubleday.

Mitchell, S. (2009). *Through the valley: The way of the cross for the end of life.* Dublin, Ireland: Veritas.

National Conference of Catholic Bishops. (1983). *Pastoral care of the sick: Rites of anointing and viaticum.* New York: Catholic Book.

O'Donohue, J. (2004). *Beauty the invisible embrace.* New York: Harper Collins.

Sulmasy, D. (2006). *The rebirth of the clinic: An introduction to spirituality in health care.* Washington: DC: Georgetown University.

Thomas, D. (2003). *Selected poems, 1934–1952.* New York: New Directions.

The Church of Christ, Scientist (Christian Science) and End-of-Life Care

Kenneth J. Doka

The Church of Christ, Scientist was founded by Mary Baker Eddy in Boston in 1879. Popularly known as Christian Scientists, the Church accepts the Bible as interpreted through Mary Baker Eddy's 1866 book *Science and Health with Key to the Scriptures*. Christian Scientists accept some core beliefs of Christianity such as the virgin birth, crucifixion, resurrection, and ascension of Jesus Christ. However, they do not view Jesus as divine, but rather as a *way-shower* sent by God as the Messiah to show the way to others. Central to Christian Science belief is that the spiritual world is good and true and that it is the only reality. The material world is false, evil, and illusionary. While the Church of Christ, Scientist does not publish membership numbers, it has acknowledged that membership has declined over the past several decades. Estimates of membership vary from 100,000 to 400,000.

SENSITIVITIES IN END-OF-LIFE CARE

While these statements reflect the official position of Christian Scientist church, it is always important to recognize that individual beliefs and practices may vary from denominational doctrine.

- *Medical Care:* Christian Scientists do not forbid members from accepting conventional medical care. However, their beliefs suggest that they should rely on prayer for healing. Focusing on the true spiritual world precludes treatment from the material world, as using conventional treatment would counteract and contradict spiritual methods. It is therefore unlikely that many Christian Scientists would seek hospice or palliative care.
- *Christian Science Practitioners and Nurses:* Christian Science practitioners are individuals trained by the Church to help and heal others by prayer according to the tenets of the Church. Christian Science nurses, also

trained by the Church, offer nonmedical care including bathing, dressing wounds, feeding, and other such services. In addition to practitioners, local branches will elect *readers* for a given period of time who lead worship. There are no ordained clergy.

- *Christian Science and Medical Care of Children:* Christian Scientists follow laws regarding the vaccination or medical treatment of children. In many states, Christian Scientists have successfully lobbied for accommodations that exempt children from medical practices such as vaccinations if objections to such practices are religiously motivated. Some states also allow the provision of spiritual healing as a defense against penalties for neglect when parents do not use conventional health care.
- *End-of-Life Ethics:* Christian Scientists can rely on their own consciences and preferences for end-of-life care.
- *Rituals:* There are no specific rituals to be performed, but it would be customary to inform a Christian Science practitioner should a Christian Scientist be admitted to a hospital or hospice. There is no specific format for funerals. If the family chooses to have a funeral service, it will likely be conducted by a Christian Science practitioner, reader, or friend of the family. Readings are likely to be from scripture or the writings of Mary Baker Eddy. While there is not generally a eulogy, the family can decide to do whatever they wish.
- *Afterlife:* Christian Science theology does not accept the belief of heaven, hell, or a judgment day. Heaven is a state of mind that seeks oneness with God while hell is a self-made anguish rooted in a belief of the material world. Death is considered illusionary. After "death," spiritual development continues.

CHAPTER 11

Orthodoxy: Theology and Ritual at the End of Life

Stanley S. Harakas

astern Orthodox Christianity, the second largest Christian Church in the Christian tradition, traces its history through an unbroken line of successive bishops to the beginnings of the Faith (i.e., to Jesus Christ and His Apostles). The Orthodox Church is a worldwide communion of local church bodies. Orthodoxy in the Americas traces its beginnings to Russian missionaries in Alaska in the early 18th century and to immigration from traditionally Orthodox nations in Eastern Europe in the early 19th century. Canonical Orthodoxy in the United States consists of nine jurisdictions using a variety of liturgical languages (including English), but sharing the same faith, liturgical practices, canonical structure, piety, spiritual ethos, pastoral practice, and ethical teachings. As such, they mutually recognize each other as belonging to one Orthodox Church. They work together not only on practical programs, such as missions, but also have entered into a process to unite the various jurisdictions into a single ecclesial body in the United States.

HUMAN LIFE AND DEATH IN ORTHODOX CHRISTIAN THEOLOGY

Many years ago, I was asked the question, "Why do people have to die physically?" Seeking to outline the traditional Orthodox perspectives on this question in a summary fashion for a popular audience, I responded:

> There are two ways, not unrelated, in which your question can be answered from the point of view of the Orthodox Christian faith. In principle, we should not die, since we were created for life, not death. But our life as creatures of God depended upon our communion with God in love and obedience. With sin, death came. The Biblical creation story says it very dramatically. "...In the sweat of your face you will eat bread till you return to the ground, for out of it you were taken: you are dust, and to dust you will return" (Genesis 3:19). More directly, the New

Testament teaches: "the wages of sin is death" (Romans 6:23). A 2nd century Father, St. Theophilos of Antioch, summed up this teaching: "So also for the man, disobedience procured his expulsion from paradise. Not, therefore, as if there were any evil in the tree of knowledge; but from his disobedience did man draw, as from a fountain, labor, pain, grief, and at last fall a prey to death" *(To Autolycus)*. Thus, because of our present fallen condition of creatureliness, our physical existence on earth comes to an end. "It is appointed for men to die once" (Hebrews 9:27).

But in a long-term sense, it has been made possible for us to overcome even physical death, while no longer standing in fear and terror of death in our present experience. The difference has come from the saving work of Christ, His death, and His victory over death through His Resurrection. (Harakas, 1987, pp. 97–98); for a fuller treatment, see Harakas, 1996, chapter 8)

The immediate conclusion arising from such an approach is that both life and death are perceived in a multidimensional way. At the least, there is spiritual life and spiritual death; physical life and physical death; temporal life and eternal life; temporal death and eternal death. Each of these has its own theological meaning and all of them are interconnected.

One way of unpacking these multiple dimensions of our topic is to look briefly at the Orthodox Dismissal Hymn for the feast of the Resurrection. Its original Greek text will be helpful in exploring the intertwined meaning of life and death in Orthodox Christian theology:

Χριστὸς ἀνέστη ἐκ νεκρόν, θανάτῳ Θάνατον πατήσας.

καὶ τοῖς ἐν τοῖς μνήμασιν, ζωὴν χαρισάμενος

There are several modern English translations used in Orthodox Churches in the United States. One of them is: "Christ is risen from the dead, by death trampling down upon Death and to those in the tombs, granting life." Clearly the themes of death and life are prominent in the hymn. In these two short lines, *dead* is used once and *death* is used twice (once in lower case and once capitalized); the word *tombs* is used once and the phrase *granting life* (ζωὴν χαρισάμενος) is used once.

The hymn is a succinct expression of what Bishop Gustav Aulen, a Lutheran theologian, described as the early Christian and continuously Eastern Orthodox understanding of the redeeming work of Jesus Christ: the *Christus Victor* theory of the Atonement (1931). Aulen describes it as the classic teaching about the saving work of Christ for humanity. It sees the human condition of sin, evil, separation from God, and both spiritual and physical death as under the dominion of the demonic forces. Because Christ took the brunt of that sin, bore evil and physical death through his death on the cross, shared in our human experience of physical death, and experienced the effects of spiritual death in others upon himself, it would have appeared that the evil had overcome good—that death had overwhelmed life. But the resurrection of Christ was the great reversal. Life, both physical and spiritual, defeats the power of death in the resurrection of Christ. Christ conquers the enemies of human existence both here in this world and in the life to come. Thus, the themes of life and death in their multiple spiritual, moral, and physical dimensions are intertwined and form important aspects of the New Testament, the writings of the Church Fathers, and the doctrinal teachings and hymnology of the Orthodox Church.

The phrase, translated "by death trampling down upon Death," is a powerful phrase. In particular, πατήσας means variously "to tread, as if to place one's foot on the neck of a defeated enemy," "to treat with contempt," "to rebut," "to do away with," and "to humble" (Lampe, 1968, p. 1050).

This Orthodox Christian theological treatment of life and death helps put the idea of end-of-life care in a context that transcends just the medical or physical dimensions of life and death. At the least, it suggests that the topic is conceived too narrowly since, theologically speaking, there is no end of life— for the grace of God grants to human life an eternal dimension. Nevertheless, even if we keep the title, we should at least modify it to be "the end of *this* life care," reserving for the future the belief in the resurrection of the body and life eternal, in which significantly for this-worldly concerns, according to the Orthodox funeral rites, "all sickness, sorrow, and sighing have fled away" (*Service Book,* 1960, p. 185).

DEATH IN THIS LIFE: PHYSICAL AND SPIRITUAL

If the focus is narrowed to death in its this-worldly dimension, there is still much that can be said theologically. Here, we can only sketch out these perspectives briefly.

Physical Death Is a Given Dimension of Earthly Life

The empirical observation that death is the lot of all human life in our present condition is affirmed by the author of the New Testament book of Hebrews who declares, "It is appointed for men to die once, and after that comes judgment" (Hebrews 9:27). From an Orthodox theological point of view, this death is neither extinction of existence, nor the end of hope, nor even of life itself.

Why God Permits Physical Death in This World

The response to this question has two dimensions. Orthodox Biblical scholar and ethicist Fr. John Breck of St. Sergius Theological Academy in Paris has succinctly articulated the Orthodox view: "To the Greek Fathers, what we inherit from Adam is not his sin and consequent guilt, but mortality. From Adam (understood, really, as an archetype), we 'inherit' the sting of death. Death has spread to all of humanity, as an inevitable consequence of our fallen nature" (Beck, 2006). Death is an inevitable aspect of our fallen created existence.

The second aspect of this question has been responded to by the Eastern and Eastern-minded Fathers of the Church by looking at the situation from the perspective of the mercy of God. Dennis Minns, in his study of the life and theology of St. Irenaeus, the second century Bishop of Lyons, describes this widespread Eastern Christian patristic view:

> As an act of mercy towards Adam and Eve, especially in view of their immaturity and inexperience, and to prevent their remaining forever disobedient adolescents, God allowed death to enter the world. Death itself was made to serve in the accomplishment of the divine plan, for, by the experience of death, humankind would learn that likeness to God was to be had as a gift from God and at the time appointed by God, and not to be seized by the earthly creature as if it had a right to it. (Minns, 1994, p. 63)

Death Is a Tragic and Wrenching Human Experience

Some have characterized Irenaeus' view as overly optimistic, a sort of kinder, gentler view of death. But the tradition also includes a more realistic—and one could say harsh, bleak, and stark—assessment of death. No one has articulated this more dramatically than St. John of Damascus in the hymns of the Orthodox funeral service, which are attributed to this eighth century Church Father. For example, in one of them he declares:

> I weep and lament when I ponder death, when I see our beauty, formed in God's image, lying in the tombs bereft of form, disfigured, without glory. O, the wonder of it! How did this mystery befall us? How were we given over to decay? How were we paired with death? Surely, as it is written, by the command of God, who gives rest to the departed. (Contos, 1995, p. 20)

Death as the Great Leveler

This realistic view of death in the theology of the Orthodox Church points to the reality that the social and material distinctions of this life are not carried on into the next. The Biblical foundation of this perspective is the parable of the rich man and Lazarus, whose condition in the next life is the opposite of their condition in this life. At the request for aid by the rich man, Abraham responds, "Son, remember that you in your lifetime received your good things, and Lazarus in like manner evil things; but now he is comforted here, and you are in anguish" (Luke 16:25). As far as the impact of death on social and economic status, St. John of Damascus' judgment is implacable:

> I called to mind the prophet, crying, "I am but dust and ashes." And I studied the tombs once more, considered the naked bones and asked myself: Now which of these was king, and which was the common soldier? Which was the rich man, which the indigent? Which man was upright and which a sinner? (Contos, 1995, p. 18)

The answers, of course, to all these questions are that social rankings after death and before the throne of God are of no importance. What is relevant is our relationship with the living God as we enter the next life.

The Certainty and Reality of Death for All Creates a Hierarchy of Values for Life

Again, the Damascene guides us to see the limited importance of the things highly valued in this life: "Where is all our attachment to worldly pursuits? Where is all the vain display of passing things? Where is the gold, where the silver? Where is the hustle and bustle of household servants? Everything is dust, ashes, shadow" (Contos, 1995, p. 18).

Nevertheless, *how we use* wealth, talents, achievements, and all this world's accomplishments is critical. When they are vehicles of spiritual and moral living, and as an expression of love for others, then they contribute to our eternal treasure (Matthew 19:21; Mark 10:21; Luke 18:22). Spiritual and moral wealth are the only possessions we can take with us into eternity. We are warned by Scripture: "Do you not know that the unrighteous will not inherit the Kingdom of God?" (1 Corinthians 6:9). For then we are living in spiritual death already. That is why the Apostle has us focus on what keeps us related to the Lord: "Whatever is true, whatever is honorable, whatever is just, whatever is pure, whatever is lovely, whatever is gracious, if there is any excellence, if there is anything worthy of praise, think about these things" (Philippians 4:8).

The Christian's Faith in the Resurrection Imbues Confidence and the Expectation of Victory Over Death

St. Paul addresses the reality of physical death that each of us faces, but unlike the philosophical existentialist who sees death as extinction, the Apostle faces death not only with peace and courage, but also with full expectation of a victorious, ongoing, unending communion with the Lord Jesus Christ.

The Christian believer faces death with confident expectation of his or her resurrection at the end times and eternal life in the Kingdom of God. St. Paul proclaims to the Christians of Corinth, "Thanks be to God, who gives us the victory through our Lord Jesus Christ. Therefore, my beloved brethren, be steadfast, immovable, always abounding in the work of the Lord, knowing that in the Lord your labor is not in vain" (1 Corinthians 15:58).

And Finally, There Is Nothing to Fear in Death for the Christian

In the fifth *Sermon on the Statues* delivered in Antioch in the mid-fourth century, St. John Chrysostom spoke to the Christians gathered there in fear of the emperor's anger. They had destroyed the imperial statues in a protest against the assessment of new taxes. Chrysostom, the master preacher, addressed their tangible anxiety at the impending threat of reprisal. They were afraid they would be punished with death for their rebellion. How confidently the Saint instructs them!

> If you are a Christian, believe in Christ! If you believe in Christ, show me your faith by your works. But how may you show this? By contempt of death! For in this we Christians differ from the unbelievers. They may well fear death, since they have no hope in the resurrection....What then is death? Just what it is to put off a garment. For the body is about the soul as a garment, and after laying this aside for a short time by means of death, we

shall resume it again with the more splendor. What is death at most? It is a journey for a season; a sleep longer than usual! So that if you fear death, you should also fear sleep!...Sorrow not for the dying man; but sorrow for him who is living in sin! (Harakas, 1987, p. 99)

As a conclusion to this section, we could note that the Orthodox Christian approach to death includes concern for dying and death, but sees them as bracketed by the human being's creation in the image of God and the spiritual task of sharing in the process of growing with the grace of God into the likeness of God as sharers in the body of Christ—His Church. Physical death then, is an aspect of our human condition, which is a transition point from this life to the next.

"END OF THIS LIFE" CARE IN THE ORTHODOX CHRISTIAN TRADITION

The Orthodox Christian tradition understands physical death as a transition from the present life to the next life with its potential for eternal communion with God or everlasting separation from God. Consequently, physical death is not as important or significant as spiritual death.

This perspective, however, does not mean that bodily and mental health and well-being are ignored or slighted in the Church's values. What follows addresses briefly and in a limited way some issues that arise from Orthodox thinking about end-of-this-life care.

Care of the Body

Since the Church holds that both soul and body are created by God so as to form together each human being, our bodies are a concrete blessing of God. "Since the body is not merely an instrument of the spirit, nor merely a dwelling place for the spirit, but a constituent part of human existence, it requires special attention for the whole person" (Harakas, 1992, p. 108). Human life, by definition, is *psychosomatic*. While the primacy is given to the soul's development and health, the body is of great importance. This means that we have a moral obligation to maintain physical health through proper nourishment, adequate exercise, and the maintenance of general good health practices. It also means that we have a moral obligation to avoid practices which abuse the body and harm its well-being. Practices such as overindulgence of alcohol, use of recreational drugs, excessive eating, or conversely, self-starvation (anorexia), ignoring the symptoms of physical disorder, and not seeking medical attention are cases of abuse of the body and are counter to the moral requirement to maintain the well-being of the body and to protect life (Harakas, 1995, p. 644).

The Therapeutic Principle

There is therefore an Orthodox Christian moral requirement that we seek to maintain our bodily health as much as we are able. We are to use both spiritual and medical means to do so. When sickness comes, it is an ethical duty, arising out of the framework of our creation in God's image, to actively seek to overcome the physical illness and to heal that which is diseased. A classic expression of this view is found in St. Basil's *Long Rules* (Basil of Cappadocia, 1962). The 55th Question, and longest in the collection, responds to an inquiry about whether or not it is appropriate for Christians to have recourse to the medical profession for treating illnesses. While enjoining spiritual healing as one way of addressing physical illness, Basil also encourages the use of medical care for healing sickness. An example of his instruction is the following: "In as much as our body is susceptible to various hurts, some attacking from without and some from within by reason of the food we eat, and since the body suffers affliction from both excess and deficiency, the medical art has been vouchsafed us by God, who directs our whole life, as a model for the cure of the soul, to guide in the removal of what is superfluous and in the addition of what is lacking" (p. 331).

Basil holds that "we must take great care to employ this medical art, if it should be necessary, not as making it wholly accountable for our state of health or illness, but as redounding to the glory of God." And elsewhere, in summary, he says, "So, then, we should neither repudiate this art altogether nor does it behoove us to repose all our confidence in it" (Basil of Cappadocia, 1962, p. 336). (For a more thorough discussion of this canon see Harakas, 1999, chapter 4.)

We could call this "the therapeutic principle." We have the moral obligation to seek appropriate means of healing of disease both for ourselves and for others in our care.

The Therapeutic Principle and End–of–This-Life Care

Given the requirement to seek healing of the illnesses of both body and mind, both on the part of the patient and on the part of healthcare providers, the first and primary concern is to do what is necessary, required, and potentially helpful to return the ill person to at least a functional level of health.

Nevertheless, a point comes when, on the basis of the knowledge and experience of the medical professionals, it becomes clear that the breakdown of the various interrelated systems of the body is irreversible. The therapeutic principle can no longer be exercised; the dying process has begun. It is precisely in this phase that the issues related to end-of-this-life care must be addressed.

While the patient is still conscious, spiritual counsel and ministrations should be offered. If a priest has been in attendance during the illness, this will come naturally. The pastoral care for the dying includes a wide range of ministries, including prayer for healing, both physical and spiritual; ministrations for comfort and strength; scriptural and other readings; counseling specifically related with dying and death; the resolution of interpersonal issues; anointing with Holy Unction or blessed oil; and the sacrament of Holy Confession and the sacrament of the Holy Eucharist. It also includes ministering to immediate family members as they face the impending death of a loved one.

However, there are also other issues that are raised when a patient enters the dying process. Many years ago I published a book of short chapters on various practical ethical concerns faced by ordinary Orthodox Christians. Among the topics treated was "Death and Dying" (Harakas, 1982, chap. 43).

Some of the perspectives presented there bear repeating in this context. Among them are the following:

- Physical death is inevitable, yet it is something which comes normally in spite of our efforts to preserve life. There is something which rings of the barbaric in calls for the elimination of human life. That is why the Orthodox Church completely and unalterably opposes euthanasia. It is a fearful and dangerous "playing at God" by fallible human beings.

- But modern medicine has perhaps gone to the other extreme. It is able now to preserve lives which God struggles to take. The various substitute mechanical organs devised by medical science are good and useful as therapeutic means. When, for instance, an artificial lung or an artificial kidney is used during an operation, it permits treatment of the diseased natural organ by the surgeon. Often, these artificial mechanical organs are used over a period of time so that the patient's life is maintained while the weakened organism is allowed time and energy to recuperate. Sometimes, such as with kidney dialysis machines and artificial lungs, almost permanent use of the machine is required. In all these cases, life is enhanced and preserved. Normally speaking, the use of such methods is a necessary and useful step in the therapeutic process whose goal is the restoration of health and life. Eventually and inevitably, however, there comes a time to die.

- Then, the body's functions break down so completely and irrevocably that these machines literally keep a dead body functioning as if it were alive. The Church holds that there comes a time to die for each of us. In fact, there is a service in the prayer book for this specific situation. When ordinary medical efforts are incapable of sustaining life, and when the body literally struggles to die, the Church prays as follows:

Thou has commanded the dissolution of the indescribable bond of soul and body, O God of Spirits, and has ordered them to be separated by Thy divine will. The body is thus to be returned to the elements from which it was made, and the soul to proceed to the source of its existence, until the resurrection of all. For this reason we implore Thee, the eternal and immortal Father, the Only-begotten Son and the All-Holy Spirit, that Thou bring about the peaceful separation of the soul of Thy servant [name] from [his or her] body.

- Here is a specific and unique situation when the church prays that life might come to an end: This decision should never be taken alone. It should be shared by the family, if possible. And, certainly, it should be made on the basis of expert medical opinion in consultation with the physician in charge of the case. It should also be made with the advice, counsel, and prayer of the priest.

To this I would like to add some pastoral reflections about the prayer mentioned above, usually referred to as "The Service or Prayer at the Tearing Away of the Soul (Εὐχὴ εἰς Ψυχορραγοῦντα)." In almost all cases where the prayer is offered, the dying patient is unconscious. I can remember only once in my pastoral ministry that a conscious dying patient requested the prayer for herself. In all other cases, the patient is deeply comatose and, essentially, struggling to die, provoking a shorter or longer "death watch" among family and friends. It is in those cases that I will, with some hesitancy and tentativeness, propose the reading of the "Prayer at the Tearing Away of the Soul." Remarkably, I have never had a family member refuse the offering of the prayer and in most cases the mere offer and the actual existence of such a prayer is a source of relief and received with gratitude. Clearly the prayer also serves to meet some spiritual needs felt by family members and others. Recently, after consulting with the husband of a dying parishioner, I also shared the decision to offer the prayer at the tearing away of the soul with two hospice nurses in attendance. They nodded appreciatively and stepped out of the room. This prayer endorses, as is often said in such cases, "letting go," and facilitates the acceptance of the death of a loved one.

"End-of-This-Life" Palliative Care

Between the beginning of the dying process and the advent of death, when the therapeutic principle can no longer be applied, palliative care designed to provide clinical comfort to the dying patient is the appropriate stance of both family and medical end-of-this-life care providers, provided spiritual and religious issues are addressed.

Palliative care ideally takes place in the home, in a family context of familiarity and love. This has become a less common practice since much palliative care still has a certain dimension of medical technology associated with it. Nevertheless, it can take place in the home, such as the last few months in the life of my own 29-year-old-daughter, Katherine Mary DeFilippo, who strongly insisted on staying at home and administering her own on-demand pain-killing medications with the help of visiting nurses and hospice personnel. To the end, she felt that somehow she was still in control of the course of her life. And as she did this, she was surrounded by a loving husband, three devoted sons, and her parents throughout that difficult and painful dying process.

In my personal and pastoral experience in the hospital setting, a patient who is in the dying process is sometimes seen as no longer of primary interest, since the mission of the medical professionals and the hospital itself is perceived as therapeutic and not palliative. For some, a dying patient represents failure.

In this regard, John and Lyn Breck, in a collaborative work on Orthodox approaches to bioethical issues, dedicate a chapter to "Care in the Final Stage of Life" that contains a fully empathetic and careful analysis of issues related to the dying process. Though there may be some still unresolved issues, this chapter generally sets a wholesome Orthodox Christian tone to the discussion (Breck & Breck, 2005, pp. 209–248).

CONCLUSION

How much and what kind of end-of-this-life care is appropriate? In the Bible, we read "The wise of heart is called a man of discernment" (Proverbs 16:21). All over the world, as well as in the most medically advanced countries such as the United States, after all therapeutic efforts fail, hundreds of people daily are mercifully allowed to go to their Maker as a result of the good judgment (discernment) of those involved. Clergy and ordinary people should leave those decisions in the hands of caring health professionals, the dying themselves (through living wills), and their closest family member, the designated caregiver. They should not let controversies swirl about them, nor should they add to them by uninformed, misplaced, inflammatory pronouncements. Rather, a spirit of quiet respect is the most appropriate, both morally and spiritually.

The basic Orthodox Christian bioethical affirmation is this: Most of the time it is right to expend every effort to fight for life, but sometimes it is right to allow death to come quietly and gently. This too, is an important and essential aspect of end-of-this-life care. The wisdom comes with knowing the difference. It was St. Paul who once said, "It is my prayer that your love may abound more and more, with *knowledge* and *all discernment*" (Philippians 1:9).

Stanley S. Harakas, *ThD, DD, is a priest of the Greek Orthodox Archdiocese of America, under the Ecumenical Patriarchate of Constantinople. He taught Orthodox Christian Ethics for 29 ½ years at Holy Cross Greek Orthodox School of Theology in Brookline, MA, retiring in 1995. He served as acting dean and dean of Hellenic College (1969–1975) and dean of Holy Cross Greek Orthodox School of Theology (1970–1980). Active in the World Council of Churches, he served on the Justice, Peace and Integrity of Creation unit. He has authored 18 books and over 150 journal and magazine articles. In 1986, he was the inaugural appointee to the Archbishop Iakovos Endowed Professorship of Orthodox Theology. Boston University honored him with the Distinguished Alumnus Award in 1986 and in 2000, Holy Cross Greek Orthodox School of Theology awarded him the honorary degree of Doctor of Divinity. He continues to write and publish in retirement.*

REFERENCES

Aulen, G. (1969). *Christus Victor: An historical study of the three main types of the idea of atonement* (A. G. Hebert, Trans.). New York: Macmillan. (Original work published 1931).

Basil of Cappadocia. (1962). *Saint Basil: Ascetical works* (M. Wagner, Trans.). Washington, DC: The Catholic University of America Press.

Breck, J. (2006). *God's righteousness.* Retrieved from http://www. orthodoxytoday.org/articles6/BreckRighteousness.php

Breck, J., & Breck, L. (2005). *Stages on life's way: Orthodox thinking on bioethics.* Crestwood, NY: St. Vladimir's Seminary Press.

Contos, L. (1995). *Sacraments and services: Book three.* Northridge, CA: Narthex Press.

Harakas, S. S. (1982). *Contemporary moral issues facing the Orthodox Christian.* Minneapolis, MN: Light and Life Publishing.

Harakas, S. S. (1987). *The Orthodox church: 455 questions and answers.* Minneapolis, MN: Light & Life Publishing.

Harakas, S. S. (1992). *Living the faith: The praxis of Eastern Orthodox ethics.* Minneapolis, MN: Light and Life Publishing.

Harakas, S. S. (1995). Eastern Orthodox Christianity. In W. T. Reich (Ed.), *Encyclopedia of Bioethics.* New York: Macmillan.

Harakas, S. S. (1996). *Health and medicine in the Eastern Orthodox tradition: Faith, liturgy, and wholeness.* Minneapolis, MN: Light and Life Publishing.

Harakas, S. S. (1999). Ethical decision-making in Saint Basil's *long rules.* In *Wholeness of faith and life: Orthodox Christian ethics.* Brookline, MA: Holy Cross Orthodox Press.

Lampe, G. H. (1968). *A patristic Greek lexicon.* Oxford: Clarendon Press.

Minns, D. P. (1994). *Irenaeus, against heresies, IV.* Washington, DC: Georgetown University Press.

Service book of the Holy Eastern Orthodox Catholic and Apostolic church (3rd ed.). (1960). Brooklyn, NY: Syrian Antiochian Orthodox Archdiocese of New York and All North America.

Jehovah's Witnesses and End-of-Life Care

Kenneth J. Doka

The Jehovah's Witnesses is a Christian denomination that differs from mainline Christianity in a number of ways including a rejection of Trinitarian beliefs. Emerging from the millennial movements of the 19th century, Jehovah's Witnesses believe that the present world order is in its last days—that Armageddon is approaching. After a climactic battle between God and Satan, earth will become a paradise for those Witnesses who survived and those who were resurrected. They believe that 144,000 will be welcomed into heaven itself. Jehovah's Witnesses have no ordained clergy and are directed by a Governing Body of Elders. They worship in Kingdom Halls. Since they view the world as corrupt and hold that Jehovah's Witnesses alone hold the truth, they tend to limit their associations with nonmembers. Baptized members who violate the basic moral principles or dispute doctrines may be shunned or *disfellowshipped* until they publicly repent. It is estimated that there are around a million members in the United States and somewhat more than a 100,000 members in Canada.

SENSITIVITIES IN END-OF-LIFE CARE

While these statements reflect the official position of the Jehovah's Witnesses, it is always important to recognize that individual beliefs and practices may vary from denominational doctrine.

- *Medical Care:* Jehovah's Witnesses accept medical and surgical treatment. However, a strong, defining belief of Jehovah's Witnesses is that they do not accept blood transfusions because they believe they are prohibited by scripture. This prohibition includes whole blood, packed red cells, plasma, white blood cells, and platelets. Preoperative autologous donation is also proscribed. Procedures that use blood fractions such as serums, hemophiliac preparations, or immune globulins or other procedures such as hemodialysis are left to the consciences of members. In cases where doctors feel compelled to get a court order mandating prohibited treatments, such as with a minor child, Jehovah's Witnesses wish to be informed and represented at court. Jehovah's Witnesses have pioneered the use of bloodless medical and surgical alternatives.

- *Hospital Liaison Committees:* In major cities and medical centers, Jehovah's Witnesses will likely have a Hospital Liaison Committee to facilitate communication between physicians, patients, and families, and assist in arranging appropriate care. In smaller communities, the Body of Elders may assume this role.
- *Advance Care Directives:* Most Witnesses will carry an advance directive that refuses blood transfusions.
- *End-of-Life Care:* Jehovah's Witnesses believe life is sacred and that the willful taking of life is prohibited. However, Jehovah's Witnesses do not believe that scripture mandates futile care that is costly and prolongs the dying process. Jehovah's Witnesses are encouraged to have advance directives that document their personal wishes.
- *Organ Donation and Transplantation:* There is no perceived scriptural objection to donation or transplantation. Such decisions can be made by individual Witnesses.
- *Autopsies:* Unless required by law, Jehovah's Witnesses generally prefer not to have autopsies performed.
- *Holidays and Birthdays:* Jehovah's Witnesses believe that all glory should be directed to Jehovah. Aside from commemorating Christ's death (around the time of Easter and Passover), they do not recognize other holidays or birthdays.
- *Dietary Issues:* While Jehovah's Witnesses will avoid eating meats that have not been drained of blood or foods such as blood sausage or soup, there are no other special dietary considerations.
- *Spiritual Care:* While Jehovah's Witnesses have no distinct rituals that are performed at the end of life, they may wish to read scriptures or pray if they are able. Members of their faith may visit to pray and read scripture. Funeral services are conducted by an Elder. They may be at Kingdom Hall, the funeral home, the home of the deceased, or the graveside. Usually brief, the services include readings and emphasize God's promised salvation and reunion.
- *Afterlife:* Jehovah's Witnesses do not believe that the soul is immortal or that there is a hell. They hope that should they die before the end time, they will be resurrected to share in paradise.

CHAPTER 12

Caring for Protestants: Asking the Right Questions

Sarah W. Nichols

Since the first rumblings of the Reformation broke out in the 1500s until the present day, the Christian Protestant movement has included a diverse stream of religious currents that has expanded into a wide and sometimes raging river of theological diversity. Ironically, these theological differences largely stem from a foundational conviction that actually binds Protestants together: a belief in what Martin Luther termed "the priesthood of all believers." This affirmation of Christ as the only intermediary needed between an individual and God, paired with Protestantism's reverence for the sole authority of Scripture, grants Protestants "the right and duty" to interpret the Scripture for themselves (Latourette, 1975, p. 715).

In this way, Protestantism's dedication to a personal relationship with God and devotion to Biblical authority have resulted in a religious movement characterized by thousands of denominations across the globe with varying interpretations of Scripture, theology, and religious practice. Protestant theology is characterized by a belief in "justification by faith," but beliefs in how salvation occurs vary greatly (Latourette, 1975, p. 715). Further, Protestants diverge widely in liturgical practice, forms of worship, and church governance. For example, the umbrella of Protestantism includes the most "high church" Anglicans, often referred to as Anglo-Catholics, whose liturgical ritual and adherence to church hierarchy are in many ways almost indistinguishable from Roman Catholicism, as well as the "undenominational" Churches of Christ, a collection of autonomous congregations that have no central headquarters or leader "other than Jesus Christ himself."

Because this theological diversity can even extend into the belief systems and practices of particular denominations, the key to providing effective end-of-life care and support to Protestant patients hinges not on having the right answers but, instead, on asking the right questions. The primary role of a caregiver is to serve as a compassionate presence to patients by connecting to them as individual human beings and responding to their particular needs and desires. Therefore, we must create a space in which we can meet patients where they are and honor their beliefs, rituals, and practices in ways that are meaningful to them. This entails our inviting them to share elements of their sacred stories of faith and religious practice, if they desire.

PROTESTANT DENOMINATIONS: AN OVERVIEW

Having a general overview of the varied Protestant denominations will enable a caregiver to better understand the religious context in which a patient's individual faith has been formed. Trying to divide the vast network of Protestant denominations into categories is difficult, but for the purposes of end-of-life care issues, this overview will delineate the following groups: mainline Protestantism, Evangelical and Fundamentalist Protestantism, Pentecostal and Charismatic Protestantism, and Anabaptist. Again, in providing effective patient care, one must realize that these abstract categories are not mutually exclusive and that there is great diversity in belief even within denominational lines.

MAINLINE PROTESTANTS

While mainline Protestant denominations vary in theology and form of governance, most share a common belief in the tenets of the Apostle's Creed that affirm "the forgiveness of sins, the resurrection of the body, and the life everlasting." As a result, while a great deal of mystery surrounds Protestant understandings of the afterlife, there is a common belief that Christians will be resurrected after death and enter into eternal life with God in Christ.

Mainline Protestants' sense of personal salvation, however, can range from a "blessed assurance" to optimistic hopefulness to vague uncertainty. Therefore, while some patients take profound comfort in the certain knowledge that when they die they are going to "a better place" to be united with God for eternity, others are fearful and questioning. Sensitive caregivers will take their cues from patients and allow them to express their feelings rather than trying to bring patients to a place of resolution.

In order to discern what might provide spiritual and emotional support to mainline Protestants, caregivers should mention options and allow patients (or their families) to identify what is meaningful to them. Most mainline Protestant denominations include more liturgy and ritual in their worship than other denominations; therefore, these patients may have a wider range of potential desires.

Protestant Communion practices include both bread and wine, although most protestant denominations use unfermented grape juice instead of wine. The exceptions to this practice are Episcopalians/Anglicans and Lutherans who customarily use wine for Communion, as well as some United Church of Christ (UCC) congregations.

Practices and Rituals

Common support practices for mainline Protestants may include being visited by a clergyperson or lay minister from their local church or denomination; having a Bible to read or Scripture read to them (the version of the Bible may be important); listening to hymns or church music; being included in a church's prayer list; being prayed for in person by a clergyperson, deacon, church elder, lay minister, or simply another Christian; receiving the laying on of hands (a form of healing prayer) by church elders or members; receiving Holy Communion from a clergyperson or lay minister, or being anointed for healing.

Common mainline Protestant denominations are listed below. The information above should provide caregivers with an idea of the kinds of resources patients might desire. Additional information to further inform caregivers is listed next to denominations with unique practices or characteristics.

American Baptist

Finding the authoritarian nature of institutional church problematic, Baptists originally formed as singular congregations to enable individuals to be in covenant relationship with God and one another. American Baptists, one of the largest Baptist associations in the United States, are typical of most Baptist denominations in their belief in the Biblical authority as the rule of life, the lordship and sacrificial work of Jesus Christ, believers' baptism of adults only by immersion, the ability of believers to be in direct relationship with God and to interpret Scripture, the independence of the local church, the church as a collection of born-again believers, and their role as Christ's witnesses in the world (Mead & Hill, 2001; American Baptist Churches, 2000). Baptists refer to the practices of baptism and the Lord's Supper as ordinances—or commands— rather than sacraments. The sermon is the central focus of the worship service and the frequency of administering the Lord's Supper generally varies from quarterly to monthly.

Sources of spiritual support to Baptist patients may include reading a Bible or devotional material (or being read to); being visited by a pastor, church deacon, or church visitor; receiving prayer or laying on of hands; or listening to recorded hymns or spiritual music.

African Methodist Episcopal (AME) Church

Born in a protest against slavery, this primarily African-American denomination is one of the world's oldest and largest Methodist bodies. As with the United Methodist Church, rather than adhering to strict doctrine, the AME Church affirms the foundational beliefs of Protestantism including recognizing baptism and Holy Communion as the two sacraments, with Communion celebrated monthly. The rise of Pentecostalism in the early 1900s brought a greater emphasis on the role of the Holy Spirit in the AME Church, which influences the emotion and joyfulness of worship.

AME Church patients may find comfort in having a Bible or devotional material to read (or being read to); being visited by a pastor or church visitor; receiving prayer or laying on of hands; or listening to hymns or spiritual music.

The Christian Church (Disciples of Christ)

The Christian Church was born out of the Reformed tradition's Campbell-Stone Restoration Movement in the 1800s in the United States. This movement was formed in response to the denominational sectarianism of the time, particularly the creedal differences that separated Christians and kept them from celebrating Holy Communion together (Piepkorn, 1978). The Christian Church attempted to reunite followers of Christ in a community that reflected New Testament faith and practices. Disciples of Christ emphasize independent, autonomous congregations and reject creeds, doctrinal statements, and church hierarchy as unscriptural (Mead & Hill, 2001). Instead, Disciples ground their beliefs in the Bible and faith in Jesus Christ as an individual's personal Lord and Savior. Disciples affirm the ordinance of "believer's baptism" by immersion only and celebrate Communion weekly, but they do not follow any common liturgical practices or orders of worship.

Disciples of Christ patients may find support in having a Bible to read (being read to), receiving prayer, listening to hymns or church music, or being visited by a minister or church member.

Episcopal Church in the U.S./Anglican

Established in the 16th century when the Church of England declared independence from Rome, Anglicanism sees itself as both *Catholic* and *Reformed*. Anglicans, primarily known as Episcopalians in the United States, affirm that they are part of "one Holy Catholic and Apostolic Church"; so, while they adopted many of the theological reforms of Protestantism, Anglican Church governance and worship remain very similar to that of Roman Catholicism. Like Roman Catholics, Anglicans view the Holy Eucharist as the central element to their Sunday worship services and a number of Anglican/ Episcopal churches offer Eucharistic services daily. Anglicans have a sacramental theology that recognizes Holy Baptism and Holy Eucharist as the two great sacraments ordained by Christ, but they also recognize five other sacramental rites: confirmation, ordination, holy matrimony, reconciliation of a penitent, and unction (anointing of the sick with oil or the laying on of hands).

In addition to the support practices and rituals listed under Mainline Protestants, Anglicans may find comfort in having a Book of Common Prayer, an Anglican book of worship and prayers; receiving Holy Eucharist (consecrated bread and wine) from a priest or lay minister; and being anointed by an Anglican/Episcopal priest. As death becomes imminent, Anglican patients and family members may want a priest to offer last rites or the Litany at the Time of Death, an end-of-life ministration offered in the Book of Common Prayer.

Evangelical Lutheran Church in America

In 1988, the culmination of decades of smaller American Lutheran denominational mergers resulted in the founding of one of the largest religious bodies in the United States, the Evangelical Lutheran Church in America (ELCA). Born out of Martin Luther's attempt to reform the Roman Catholic Church in the 16th century, Lutheranism emphasizes the sole authority of the Bible while also affirming its continuity with the history and identity of the Catholic past (Piepkorn, 1978). ELCA members recognize Holy Baptism and Holy Eucharist as the church's two sacraments and hold them to be channels of God's grace and presence. In recent years, many Lutheran congregations have been moving from the predominant monthly celebration of Holy Communion to a weekly Eucharistic service.

In addition to having a Bible to read, receiving prayer, or being visited by a pastor or church member, Lutheran patients may want to receive Holy Eucharist (consecrated bread and wine) or be anointed by a Lutheran pastor.

Presbyterian (USA)

The Presbyterian Church is part of the stream of Reformed churches that trace their roots back to Zurich, Geneva, and Scotland (Piepkorn, 1978).

Presbyterians adhere to the Reformation doctrine that firmly grounds church identity in the local community of professing Christians instead of in a hierarchical clerical order. Presbyterians affirm the primacy of Scripture and look to written "Confessions" to provide the central tenets of Reformed faith and guide members in discerning Scripture (Small, 2006). As a result of the Liturgical movement in the late 20th century, Presbyterians embraced a more ecumenical form of worship by recognizing the Christian liturgical year and embracing liturgies and rituals reflective of the early church (Piepkorn, 1978). Many congregations began increasing the frequency of Communion from quarterly to monthly or, for a minority, even weekly.

Presbyterian patients may find comfort in having a Bible to read (or being read to); receiving prayer; being visited by a minister, deacon, or elder; and, perhaps, receiving the Lord's Supper.

Society of Friends/Quakers

Founded by George Fox in the 17th century, Quakerism emphasizes the experiential aspects of relationship with God and maintains that God's revelations continue in the present day. Friends believe that the "Inner Light" of God resides in every human being and that the responsibility of ministry rests on all believers, making clergy unnecessary. Quakers are nonliturgical and, because they hold all of life to be sacramental, Friends do not celebrate sacramental rituals such as Baptism or the Lord's Supper. While Friends value the Bible, they place great importance in fostering present experiences with God both individually and communally, such as by listening in silence. Their beliefs lead them to be service-oriented, anti-war, and to affirm the equality of all people.

Patients who are Friends would likely feel supported by the presence of other Quakers, as well as having materials for religious reflection, such as Scripture, poetry, or Quaker publications.

United Church of Christ/Congregationalists

The United Church of Christ (UCC) came into being in 1957 as part of the Ecumenical movement when the Evangelical and Reformed Church merged with the Congregational Christian Churches. Because the United Church of Christ comes from the Reformed tradition of "confessing churches," the UCC does not adhere to creeds as authoritative, and their statement of faith is "regarded as a testimony, and not as a test of faith" (Small, 2006). Local churches are autonomous, and the UCC identity and mission is grounded in its present witness of the Gospel rather than in traditions or confessions of the past. The UCC recognizes baptism and the Lord's Supper as the two sacraments of the church but does not have specific doctrinal statements about either (Piepkorn, 1978). The frequency of Communion varies, but is monthly in most congregations.

UCC patients may find comfort in having a Bible to read, receiving prayer, being visited by their minister or church visitor, and, perhaps, receiving Communion.

United Methodist Church

The 20th century brought significant reunification to American Methodism, culminating in 1968 when the United Methodist Church was formed. Methodism is rooted in two Christian traditions: Anglicanism, influenced by John and Charles Wesley's Methodist movement of the 1700s, and German Reformed Pietism. The United Methodist Church does not espouse specific theology and doctrine but, instead, emphasizes the foundational beliefs of Protestantism and articulates doctrinal standards to inform church practice. Following John Wesley's call to "practical divinity," United Methodists emphasize the importance of God's grace and its influence on Christian living. Methodists recognize two sacraments: baptism and Communion. Infant and adult baptism is practiced, usually by sprinkling, and the frequency and manner of Communion varies.

Pastoral care to support Methodist patients may include having a Bible or devotional material to read; being visited by a pastor or church member; receiving prayer; listening to hymns or church music; or, perhaps, receiving Holy Communion.

EVANGELICAL AND FUNDAMENTALIST PROTESTANTS

Protestants who self-identify as evangelical or fundamentalist are by no means monolithic in their beliefs, worship styles, or practices. However, they do tend to hold the following beliefs in common: the inerrancy of the Bible; being born again (receiving personal salvation by accepting Christ as one's Lord and Savior); and, an evangelical commitment to sharing the good news with others so that they may also be saved rather than spending eternity in hell. For evangelicals and fundamentalists, the impact of the fall of humanity in the Garden of Eden informs both their conviction of the need for personal redemption and their requirement to oppose the ongoing reality of sin and evil in the world. Evangelicals and fundamentalists largely focus on teaching and preaching, with little to no liturgy or ritual in their worship.

Many evangelical and fundamentalist Protestants hold their church's Christian beliefs as the central guiding principle in their lives. These patients will tend to be clear about their belief system. A particularly sensitive situation can occur when a patient's family is evangelical or fundamentalist and family members are unsure if the patient is "saved" or not. In these situations, a caregiver must be responsive to the wishes of the patient and respect his or her boundaries while also honoring the family's belief system. The role of women in evangelical and fundamentalist churches usually does not include ordination or positions of leadership, such as teaching men, so some patients may not be open to a female chaplain.

Practices and Rituals

As always, it is critical to discern the patient's individual desires; however, for the most part, evangelical and fundamentalist patients tend to have common sources of spiritual support. Having a Bible to read or being read the Bible is often of great comfort and may also provide spiritual strength. In many cases, the patient may have a particular version of the Bible that is preferred. Receiving prayer, specifically the laying on of hands by a minister or church elders, is usually an integral part of religious practice for someone who is sick or dying. Further, being placed on a list to receive ongoing prayer by church members or prayer groups (sometimes referred to as *prayer vigils*) may be a source of support to a patient. Most patients will want to be visited by clergy or church members. Some may want to listen to hymns or praise songs for spiritual sustenance.

Churches of Christ

The Stone-Campbell Restoration Movement of the American 19th century gave birth to the Christian Church (Disciples of Christ) from which the churches of Christ split in the early 20th century. The churches that sprang from the Restoration Movement were founded in an effort to break with past influences that had shaped and, they believed, corrupted the Church and to attempt to re-establish the Church of the first century (Foster, 2006). As a result, the autonomous congregations identified as churches of Christ reject all Christian creeds and liturgical practices as accretions that depart from the purity of early Christianity. Instead, they believe that people can read the New Testament and discern the simple facts of the Christian faith for themselves. They disallow organs and other instruments during worship, and, like the first century Church, they observe the memorial of the Lord's Supper on a weekly basis. They believe the only pardon available for human sinfulness is faith in Christ, repentance, confession, and baptism by immersion. The churches of Christ do not identify as a denomination because they feel that the notion fails to honor Christ as the sole head of the Church and obstructs Christian unity.

Churches of Christ patients would likely find comfort and support in having a Bible or church sermons to read (being read to); being visited by a minister, church elder, or deacon; and receiving prayer. Because churches of Christ sing a cappella in worship services, listening to recorded instrumental hymns may not be appropriate.

Church of the Nazarene

The Church of the Nazarene is one of the largest denominations to come out of the Holiness Movement of the 1860s and, therefore, could also be included with Pentecostal/Charismatic denominations. However, Nazarene theological roots are Wesleyan/Methodist, and church practice focuses more on lifestyle than on the role of the Holy Spirit. In keeping with Holiness church tradition, Nazarene doctrine advocates sanctification as a second work of grace that comes after a believer's justification through repentance and faith in Christ. This doctrine of believer's sanctification is central to Nazarene faith, required of leaders, and reflected in the church's call for members to lead sanctified lives, including abstaining from alcohol or tobacco, forbidding gambling or participation in lotteries, refraining from membership in societies that require oath-taking, and rejecting some forms of popular entertainment and culture (Piepkorn, 1978; Mead & Hill, 2001). Nazarenes affirm two sacraments: Communion and baptism, which is for believers but is allowed for young children. While Nazarenes believe in divine healing, they regularly use medical facilities for treatment.

Nazarene patients may find spiritual support in being visited by church leadership or members, receiving prayer, or having a Bible or devotional material to read.

Lutheran, Missouri Synod

The Lutheran Church–Missouri Synod, the second largest Lutheran denomination in the United States, finds its roots in the 19th century German immigration into the United States (Mead & Hill, 2001). More congregational than other Lutheran bodies, Missouri Synod Lutherans emphasize the inerrancy of Scripture and the centrality of Lutheran confessional statements. Missouri Synod Lutherans recognize baptism and the Lord's Supper as the two sacraments. While the practice of celebrating the Lord's Supper weekly has been increasing in recent years, the majority of parishes offer Holy Communion twice a month (Wieting, n.d.).

In addition to having a Bible to read, receiving prayer, or being visited by a pastor or church member, Lutherans of the Missouri Synod may want to receive Holy Communion.

Presbyterian Church in America

The Presbyterian Church in America (PCA) was formed in 1973 by conservative Presbyterians who withdrew from the Presbyterian Church, U. S., largely due to differences over the authority of the Bible, social and doctrinal issues, and the ordination of women (Mead & Hill, 2001). The PCA affirms the inerrancy of scripture, uses the Westminster Confession of Faith as its doctrinal standard, and recognizes baptism and the Lord's Supper as sacraments. The frequency of the Lord's Supper varies from congregation to congregation but ranges from quarterly to monthly.

PCA patients may find comfort in having a Bible or devotional material to read, receiving prayer, listening to hymns or church music, or being visited by a pastor or church officer.

Southern Baptist Convention

The Southern Baptist Convention is made up of autonomous Southern Baptist congregations that believe in the inerrancy of Scripture, the importance of personal repentance and faith for salvation, believer's baptism by immersion only, and the importance of evangelism and missions. Southern Baptists emphasize teaching and evangelism. The ordinance of the Lord's Supper ranges in frequency from quarterly to monthly among congregations.

Southern Baptist patients would likely find comfort in having a Bible, sermons, or devotional materials to read (being read to); being visited by a minister, church elder, or deacon; receiving prayer; or listening to hymns or Christian music.

PENTECOSTAL AND CHARISMATIC PROTESTANTS

While there are large American and worldwide Pentecostal and charismatic denominations, there are thousands more small Pentecostal denominations in the United States, as well as many Pentecostal or charismatic congregations that are not affiliated with a national church. Additionally, many mainline denominations include a small percentage of congregations that have been part of the "charismatic movement" and whose members self-identify as charismatic.

While their theology is similar to that of evangelicals and fundamentalists, Pentecostal and charismatic Protestants have a greater focus on the ongoing role of the Holy Spirit. Manifestations of the presence and power of the Spirit working in the lives of the people of God are important aspects of Pentecostal life and worship. They believe that spiritual gifts, such as speaking in tongues, words of wisdom, and miraculous healings, are spread throughout the community of faithful believers to be used to build up the body of Christ and to glorify God. Churches in the Holiness branch of Pentecostalism believe that Christians are "set apart" to participate in Christ's "divine mission" and that the Holy Spirit's presence in the heart of Christians both sanctifies them and inspires holy Christian living (Stafford, 2001, p. 27). Pentecostal Christians engage in spiritual warfare to fight the power of Satan at work in the world and are committed to the laying on of hands and praying for healing. Pentecostal worship is often exuberant and emotional, including great joy and laughter as well as tears.

Pentecostals believe that all Christians will be with God for eternity. When Christ returns, Christians who are alive will be raptured to meet the Lord in the air. Those Christians who have died will be raised from their graves to be "caught up together" with Christ and his faithful. Therefore, Pentecostal Christians have the comfort of knowing that they will always be with the Lord.

Practices and Rituals
Pentecostal/Charismatic Protestant patients may find comfort in being visited by a pastor or church leader and receiving prayer, specifically the laying on of hands, as well as receiving ongoing prayer by church members or through prayer vigils. Sources of support may also include having a Bible to read or being read to, listening to praise music, or being surrounded by church members and friends.

Assemblies of God
The Assemblies of God, the largest Pentecostal denomination, is a group of churches and assemblies that united as a body in 1914 while still retaining their independence as local congregations. They follow the ordinances of baptism and the Lord's Supper. For Assemblies of God members, the baptism of the Holy Spirit can usually be identified by the gift of speaking in tongues. Patient supports are listed in Practices and Rituals above.

Church of God in Christ

The Church of God in Christ stresses the importance of receiving the sanctifying power of the Holy Spirit to live a holy, sanctified life (Mead & Hill, 2001). Baptism of the Spirit is evidenced by speaking in tongues and the gift of healing. They recognize the ordinances of baptism by immersion, the Lord's Supper, and foot washing. Patient supports are listed in Practices and Rituals above.

ANABAPTIST

Mennonite

Coming to the United States in waves starting in the late 17th century, Mennonites maintain the Anabaptist focus on the importance of Godly living, as reflected in the Sermon on the Mount, rather than on theology or liturgy (Mead & Hill, 2001). Mennonite beliefs include a commitment to nonviolence, refusal to take oaths, the use of church discipline to hold standards of faith and practice, and the importance of living a Christian life as a testimony of redeemed discipleship (Piepkorn, 1978). Mennonites operate as autonomous congregations with, primarily, self-supporting ministers who have secular employment (Mead & Hill, 2001). Mennonites partake of the Lord's Supper either twice a year or monthly, sometimes including foot washing in those services as well. Baptism is for believers only and occurs by pouring. Mennonites are known for caring for the needs of church members as well as for their international relief and justice efforts.

Mennonite or other Anabaptist patients would likely find comfort in being visited by church members, receiving prayer, or having a Bible to read.

Rev. Sarah W. Nichols, an ordained Episcopal priest, serves as director of pastoral care for The Episcopal Home Communities, a nonprofit corporation that operates three continuing care retirement communities in southern California. As director of pastoral care, Rev. Nichols oversees the communities' chaplains, supports the spiritual well-being of residents, families, and staff, and provides training in compassion fatigue, palliative care, and end-of-life issues. She participated in the 2007 ACE Project: Advocating for Clinical Excellence Transdisciplinary Palliative Care Training and served as a panelist in the two subsequent ACE conferences. In 2009, she was one of 40 doctors, psychologists, chaplains, and spiritual care professionals who took part in the "Improving the Quality of Spiritual Care as a

Dimension of Palliative Care Project" as part of the National Consensus Project for Quality Palliative Care. She was a speaker at the California Association of Long Term-Care Medicine 2010 Annual Meeting.

REFERENCES

American Baptist Churches. (2000). *10 facts you should know about American Baptists.* Available at: http://www.abc-usa.org/portals/0/ABC10FactsBrochure.pdf

Foster, D. A. (2006). The nature of the apostolicity of the church: Perspectives from churches of Christ. In T. A. Campbell, A. K. Riggs, & G. W. Stafford (Eds.), *Ancient faith and American-born churches: Dialogues between Christian traditions.* Mahwah, NJ: Paulist Press.

Kinnamon, M. (2006). The place of an authoritative teaching office in the Christian Church (Disciples of Christ). In T. A. Campbell, A. K. Riggs, & G. W. Stafford (Eds.), *Ancient faith and American-born churches: Dialogues between Christian traditions.* Mahwah, NJ: Paulist Press.

Latourette, K. S. (1975). *A history of Christianity* (vol. 2). San Francisco: Harper San Francisco.

Mead, F. S., & Hill, S. S. (2001). *Handbook of denominations in the United States* (11th ed.) C. D. Atwood (Ed.). Nashville, TN: Abingdon Press.

Piepkorn, A. C. (1978). *Profiles in belief: The religious bodies of the United States and Canada.* San Francisco: Harper and Row.

Small, J. D. (2006). Confessing the faith in the Reformed tradition. In T. A. Campbell, A. K. Riggs, & G. W. Stafford (Eds.), *Ancient faith and American-born churches: Dialogues between Christian traditions.* Mahwah, NJ: Paulist Press.

Stafford, G. W. (2001). The holiness perspective on reconciling love in worship. In T. A. Campbell, A. K. Riggs, & G. W. Stafford (Eds.), *Ancient faith and American-born churches: Dialogues between Christian traditions.* Mahwah, NJ: Paulist Press.

Wieting, K. (n.d.). *The Lord's Supper on the Lord's Day.* Retrieved July 14, 2010, from http://www.lcms.org/pages/internal.asp?NavID=809

The Church of Jesus Christ of Latter-Day Saints and End-of-Life Care

Kenneth J. Doka

The Church of Jesus Christ of Latter-Day Saints (LDS), popularly known as the Mormon Church, was founded by Joseph Smith in 1830. The term *Mormon* was originally used derisively but it is now embraced by members of the LDS church. While Mormon refers to all who adhere to the belief system expounded by Smith, most Mormons belong to The Church of Jesus Christ of Latter-Days Saints, though there are some independent, fundamentalist groups. Other groups, which divided from the LDS church after Smith's death in 1844, such as the Community of Christ (formally known as the Reorganized Church of Jesus Christ of Latter-Day Saints, or RLDS) would prefer not to be called Mormons. Mormons consider themselves a distinct branch of Christianity (along with Catholic, Protestant, and Orthodox Christians). In addition to the Old and New Testament, Mormons accept the *Book of Mormon* as divinely inspired and believe that God still speaks through revelation. The LDS church is headquartered in Salt Lake City, Utah. The Church has around 13 million members throughout the world; slightly less than 50% live in the United States.

SENSITIVITIES IN END-OF-LIFE CARE

While these statements reflect the official position of The Church of Jesus Christ of Latter-Day Saints, it is always important to recognize that individual beliefs and practices may vary from denominational doctrine.

- *Dietary:* Members are expected to abstain from alcohol, illegal drug use, coffee, tea, and tobacco, and they generally avoid caffeine products. While meat can be eaten, there is an emphasis on a healthy diet that focuses on grains and vegetables.
- *Spiritual Care:* LDS members generally prefer to be connected to local LDS congregations rather than be served by a non-LDS chaplain. Mormons do

have rituals involving illness such as prayer and anointing with oils that should be conducted by someone with priesthood authority.

- *Medical Decisions:* When facing end-of-life decisions, LDS members study scripture, pray for revelation, and consult with their bishop and other members. They would be open to consultation with expert medical opinion. While holding that God can work miracles and heal, members of the LDS church fully accept the blessings of conventional medicine.
- *End-of-Life Ethics:* Death is considered a natural aspect of life. Mormons need not accept care that prolongs life but they should not do anything to actively hasten death. Individual ethical decisions should involve consultation with LDS bishops.
- *Autopsies and Organ Donations:* These are individual decisions for families.
- *Funeral Rituals:* Funerals for members of the LDS church are open to Mormons and nonmembers. Funeral rituals will usually include viewings, a service at the Temple or funeral home chapel, a graveside service, and a shared meal. Prayers, scriptures, hymns, remembrances, and eulogies may be incorporated into the service. Services may be long—perhaps 2–3 hours. Burial is generally preferred over cremation.
- *Afterlife:* Members of the LDS church believe that souls are immortal. After death, spirits go to a spirit world to await a physical resurrection. This time still allows for growth and instruction. Those who still do not repent face an eternal hell. Non-Mormons who lead worthy lives will receive a reward in the afterlife but will not live in the presence of God. Mormons will baptize the dead as a way to ensure that familial relationships continue in the afterlife.

CHAPTER 13

Islamic Spirituality and End-of-Life Care: Guidelines for Chaplains and Counselors

Yahya Hendi

Islam is the religion of about 1.3 billion people around the world. Close to 7 million of those are Americans. Muslims believe that this world was founded by a higher power; in Arabic, they call him *Allah*, which is the word for the very God found in Jewish and Christian scriptures. God is the creator of this world and the one worthy of worship, devotion, and love. The belief in God is called *Tawhid,* referring to the oneness of God. The one and only God is referred to in many ways in liturgy, prayers, and Muslim meditations. The most commonly used divine attributes are the Loving, the Almighty, the Merciful, the Compassionate, the Healer, and the Most Just.

Muslims believe that Islam was revealed to Prophet Muhammad, who was born in 570 and died in 632. Prophet Muhammad's exemplary life practices and sayings are referred to by the words *Sunnah* or *Hadith*, often called the second most important body of literature after the Qur'an. Muslims believe the Qur'an to be the divine revelation God sent to Muhammad as a confirmation of what was revealed in earlier revelations to Jesus and Moses but with a new focus on morality and ethics. While prophecy guides us to travel towards God, revelation is expected to prepare Muslims to return back to God in a way pleasing to the Most High. While the Qur'an offers, word for word, God's most important teaching for Muslims, Hadith represents the prophet's interpretations of the scriptures and detailed data regarding Islamic theology, creed, and ethics.

Islam offers its followers an understanding of the concept of God, life, and salvation and gives different interpretations of human experiences in this world. It attempts to answer the questions: Why are we created and why do we live, rejoice, and suffer? What is life and death and how do we deal with end-of-life experiences? This chapter will focus on one element in human life: spirituality and theology of life, suffering, illness, and death.

LIFE AND DEATH

Human beings have no choice but to return to God. Everyone does, and everyone will meet God. However, some people go happily with the knowledge that they have submitted to the instructions brought by prophets and that God does not break his promise to reward them. Others will pay the price for their failure to do so.

The Qur'an makes it clear that death is inescapable. It is the final stage in the life of all living things including human beings. "Every soul shall taste death" (3:185). "Surely death, from which you flee, shall encounter you. Then you shall be taken back to the knower of all things" (62:8).

Life in this world is not an absolute life and it cannot be depended on in any way because it lasts a short time. So also, death at the end of life is not an absolute death. Rather, it is a transferal from one mode of existence into another, called the grave, where things continue to happen and where the dead person continues to have experiences. Experiences are attributes of living beings, not dead things. Hence, this is a death in relation to this world, not in relation to the whole of reality.

God is called in Islam "The Alive" and "The Self-Subsistence." In other words, God only is alive through God's self and subsists through God's self. Tawhid demands that nothing is alive but God. Every thing other than God is dead in relation to God. Therefore, if things have so-called life, it is because God gave them life. If God gives life, it is also he who takes it. When the Qur'an speaks of death, it speaks of it in relation to this world, and it is only God who decides when this can happen.

DEATH AND DYING

Suicide is forbidden in Islamic ethics. There is a direct and explicit text in the Qur'an and Hadith on the issue of suicide. Two very well known Qur'anic verses speak to this issue: "And do not cast yourselves into destruction" (2:195) as well as "And kill not yourselves" (4:29). According to Islamic creed, God is the creator of the human life; therefore, a person does not own his or her life and hence cannot terminate it.

Resurrection and judgment are central in the divine scheme for humans. The nature of the future life of a person depends on his or her performance in this life, in the span between birth and death—or, more accurately, between adulthood and death. For the Qur'an, the afterlife is as concrete and palpable as the life in this world. There is a natural continuity between the two and death is the passage between them. The Qur'an continually emphasizes the unlimited mercy and forgiveness of God, but it links a person's future with his or her performance here on earth in addition to the grace of God Most High.

As for intercession, the Qur'an raises the issue several times but seems to deny it for fellow human beings. God's grace, Prophet Muhammad, and the deeds of a good person are the only ones offering intercession for the dead in the life to come. God's mercy may allow some to intercede out of God's divine love for some.

The dead person does not have to await the Day of Judgment to receive rewards and punishments but begins his or her reckoning in the grave. The doors of the heavens are opened to the deceased in accordance with their desserts while they are yet in the grave. The intermediary stage, *Barzakh*, starts right after burial.

The entirety of the Qur'an is directed toward inculcating in human beings a sense of piety or moral responsibility called *Taqwa*, which literally means to protect oneself against moral peril. Taqwa is an instrument or an inner power that enables one to discriminate between right and wrong and to judge one's own actions. On the Day of Judgment, deeds will be weighted and passed on to his or her final destiny.

Death for Islam, then, is a mere link or a passage between two segments of a continuous life: "God receives the souls when they die and those who do not die God receives them in their sleep; God then keeps those for whom He has decreed death while others He releases until the appointed term." (Qur'an 39:42) This transition or passage of death is portrayed by the Qur'an as being a difficult experience for the wicked, probably because they did not believe in an afterlife or did not prepare for it. The only life they knew was coming to an end and this they spent it in evil-mongering.

God will judge with justice and every human being will be paid in full for what they have done. Therefore, one must be ready for that stand in the divine court to be questioned about his or her decisions, behaviors, and actions. Nothing can be hidden and death is the path to that assured end.

WHEN DEATH NEWS IS PRONOUNCED

When a person is dying, relatives and close friends are normally present because Islam recognizes no intermediaries between humans and God. It has, strictly speaking, no clergy. Yet, many may choose to ask for Imams or Muslim chaplains to be present at the moment of, or immediately following, death.

In general, though, anyone knowledgeable of the faith may perform certain administering sacraments. Those may include:

1. Asking the dying person to recite the *shahadah*, or testimony of faith: "There is no God but the Almighty Creator and Muhammad is a messenger of God." The person may do it on behalf of the dying person only when the dying person cannot do it.

2. Uttering the following statement may be helpful: "Allah, God the Almighty, is great."

3. Saying the following prayers may also help: "Oh God! I ask You for a perfect faith, a sincere assurance, a reverent heart, a remembering tongue, a good conduct of recommendation, and a true repentance, a repentance before death, rest at death, and forgiveness and mercy after death, clemency at the reckoning, winning paradise and escape from fire, all by Your mercy. O Mighty One, O forgiver, Lord, increase me in knowledge and join me unto good. O God may the end of my life be the best of it, may my closing acts be my best acts and may the best of days be the day when I shall meet You. Amen."

4. When the patient has breathed his or her last breath, their eyes should be gently closed and the following prayers recited on the deceased's behalf: "O God! Make [his or her] death light for [him or her], and render easy what [he or she] is going to face after this, and bless [him or her] with Your support and make [his or her] new abode better for [him or her] than the one he has left behind. Amen."

Usually, if the deceased has done wrong to someone or has failed to pay a debt, the forgiveness of that person of the deceased is sought because according to Islamic theology, the fulfillment of the rights of fellow people has priority over the rights of God, and God will not forgive violations of humans rights unless those wronged have forgiven.

FUNERALS

Islam encourages attending funeral services as a meritorious act whether those who participate in the services personally knew the deceased or not. Indeed, many services may be held at the same time in different places for the same person. The funeral service is considered spiritually beneficial both for the dead and for those who participate in the services. The Islamic tradition enjoins burial of the dead without unnecessary delay. Burial rites are simple and austere. Wailing loudly for the dead is forbidden, yet grief and sadness are acceptable. However, patience is expected to be observed.

When entering the cemetery, one should recite a special greeting to the deceased ones by saying: "Peace be upon all of you, all people of graves!" One should be silent and use this time for personal reflections and self-examination. The graves are dug on a southeast–northwest line. The head of the deceased is directed toward northwest in the United States, for that is the direction of the five daily prayers—toward the city of Mecca. Bodies are expected to be laid on the soil and dust.

ILLNESS AND SUFFERING AS A PART OF LIFE

Perfection belongs to God alone. This life, when compared to God, is spoken of as a lowly imperfect world full of imperfections. Yet God governs this world by His divine mercy, love, and justice. If that is the case, then why suffer with illness and death? Is illness and death a punishment from God or a consequence of His wrath? Or is it a fact of human life as we know it?

According to the Qur'an, diseases are neither divine punishment nor a consequence of the wrath of God. Sometimes humans are tested by sickness or affliction such as loss of wealth and death. Also according to the Qur'an, the adversities of life—physical illness being one of them—are merely a part of the human life that one must expect. Learning to deal with them is a matter of religious practice. "It is God who created me and it is He who guides me, who gives me food and drink and when I am ill, it is He who heals me. He is the One who will cause me to die and then bring me back to life. He is the one I hope will forgive my mistakes on the day of Judgment" (Qur'an 26:78–82).

Illness is not a consequence of sin since one can point to many innocent babies and children with severe and incurable illnesses. The Qur'an does not see illness to be due to the wrath of God since many of God's beloved creatures also suffer. Their patience is also praised. "And Job when he cried out to his Lord: 'Adversities have seized me while You are the most merciful.' I, God responded to him and removed the adversity he was facing" (Qur'an 21:83). "I, God, found Job very patient. How excellent was such a worshipper" (Qur'an 38:44).

In fact, what matters is the manner in which one handles adversities and suffering:

> I shall test you with a bit of fear and hunger, plus a shortage of wealth, lives and products. Give glad tidings to those who patiently persevere and to who say, whenever some misfortune strikes them, "To God we belong and to Him we will return" (Qur'an 2:156-157).

In another verse: "And to be firm and patient in pain or suffering and adversity and through all periods of panic, such are the people of truth, the God loving" (Qur'an 2:177).

The quality of a true believer must continue to be the same. Anyone suffering an illness should remain patient, for there is no reward better or more enriching than that reserved for those who endure in patience. "How remarkable is the case of the believer! There is good for him in everything. When he receives good, he is grateful to God and hence, rewarded. When he is afflicted with a calamity, he is patient hence, rewarded" (Hadith collection).

Illness acts as a purifying process if the ill person exercises patience. The prophet Muhammad is said to have said, "God purifies His worshippers with diseases and poverty as fever sheds the sins of a year in one night." God is also in touch with the ill and the suffering as "He answers the prayers of patient, sick persons." Such feeling gives the sick person the ultimate hope for being connected directly with the ultimate source of healing and power.

If the suffering person, the sick, and the dying are that close to God, Islam encourages Muslims neither to ignore nor to abandon the need of those individuals. Prophet Muhammad said: "Visit the sick and the dying ones and ask them to pray for you as their prayers are accepted and their cries are heard by God." It is, indeed, an Islamic moral etiquette to visit the sick and the dying ones as a way of providing them with moral and physical support, but also to be in the presence of the divine with them. Muhammad said: "A caller from heaven calls out to the person who visits a sick and dying person, 'You are good and your path is good. May you enter your residence in paradise in peace.'" It is also recommended that one prays for the recovery and good health of the ill and urge him or her to endure their pain patiently.

God recognizes our human nature. Therefore, it is permitted for patients to complain of pain and illness to physicians or friends, provided they do not do so to express their anger or impatience with God. Maintaining good faith will result in rewards for the ill for all the good deeds he or she would usually perform in a state of health.

Islam does not want us to waste our resources by trying to find the philosophical reasons behind physical illness or suffering since it is regarded as a fact of life and a passage to eternity. It directs our efforts to cope with illness and seek a cure. Muslims are taught to seek medical and technological advances to find a way out of suffering, but only as a gift from God. One should seek cures for illness, but only with the belief that God grants such cures.

Prophet Muhammad said, "Look for the cures of your diseases as God has not sent a disease for which he has not sent a cure."

SOME SUPPLICATIONS USED BY MUSLIM PATIENTS

"O God! The Sustainer of the universe. Remove my illness and cure my disease. You are the One who cures. No other one can cure or gives permission to cure but you. Grant me a cure that leaves no sickness."

"I seek refuge in God, the powerful Lord, from the evils of pain."

"O God! I ask for Your guidance as you are the All-knowledgeable, the All-powerful, the almighty. You are capable and I am not. You know and I do not. You know that this thing I am faced with is good for my faith and my sustenance and for my hereafter, then ordain it for me and make it easy on me to deal with. God if you know that is good neither for my souls not my flesh take it away from me and protect me from it. Lord You are the One to ask to send patience in to my heart and in my life."

QUR'ANIC TREATMENT OF HEALING

The Qur'an says, "And we reveal of the Qur'an that which is a healing and a mercy for believers" (17:82). This verse reflects the Qur'anic definition on illness and healing. The teachings of the Qur'an attempt to deal with the human being as a whole—body, heart, and soul. The Qur'an suggests that the healing process must deal with all aspects of the human being that secular medicine has failed to do.

The Qur'an contains teachings related to personal behavior, attitudes, and dealings that guide the individual in the conduct of his or her daily affairs. It also contains teachings that deal with general matters of society and which, if applied correctly, will lead to the achievement of general goals such as freedom, justice, and improved economic conditions. All of these teachings lead to the making of a balanced, emotionally stable, and successful individual who is able to make better decisions and realize better achievements in life. Such an individual will enjoy a much higher degree of well-being and, as a result, better emotional health, a better immune system, and a healthier physical condition. Negative emotions are the greatest enemy of the immune system.

Negative emotions can manifest in various ways: frustration, depression, grief, helplessness, hopelessness, anger, hate, desire of revenge, feelings of guilt, fear, anxiety, worry, insecurity, or any combination of these. The effect on the immune system can result in a variety of immune deficiencies or dysfunctions. Once the immune system fails to function properly, all types of physical illnesses can develop.

The Qur'an first makes it clear to its readers that negative emotions are undesirable and very harmful. The Qur'an then gives them clues as to how to get rid of them. The Quar'an teaches: "Do not fear." "Do not despair." "Do not keep angry." "Seek refuge in God from helplessness and laziness."

The Qur'an suggests that people should act in light of the following factors:

1. What may cause negative emotions is not going to disappear. Since perfection is for God alone, everybody else and everything else is imperfect or deficient.

2. There is another list: the list of good things and emotions in humans. Since all good things are from God the Almighty, we can call this a list of blessings. What happens if I look at the list of blessings? I feel cheerful and grateful. When I feel good, my efficiency and productivity improves. When I feel grateful, I do good deeds to express my gratitude, and the list of blessings grows longer, from good to better.

3. If I focus my eyes on a certain object, it is impossible to focus my eyes or attention on another object at the same time. This means that if I focus on the list of blessings, not only will I feel cheerful and grateful with improved performance and immune function, but I will also not be able to see the bad list clearly. Once the bad list fades out of my site, the depression and related miserable emotions disappear too.

Does this mean that one should never look at the bad list and have a bad feeling? Not at all. As a matter of fact, one should be properly looking at the bad list several times a day—every time something bad happens. But after a few moments, I should return my sight and attention to the list of blessings.

The Qur'an achieves its healing and health-promoting effect by utilizing three approaches:

The legal approach is through prohibitions against matters hazardous to health (e.g., disbelief, alcohol, excessive eating, etc.) and by enjoining matters that promote health (e.g., prayers, fasting, ablution, bathing, and breastfeeding). This legislation has a direct impact on the health of the individual.

The guiding approach is through the provision of general rules and regulations that guide the individual through the conduct of his or her daily affairs. The guidance approach has an indirect positive effect on the heath and well-being of the individual.

The third approach is though the direct healing effect of the Qur'an on the various organs of the body, which is called *Ruqia*. It is important to remember that even though utilizing the Qur'an will render us better able to deal with, tolerate, and control illness, illness itself will not be completely eliminated.

Illness provides a challenge to the affected person to find the cure. Thus, illness may be viewed as: a way of gaining forgiveness of one's sins; an investment in rewards for the one suffering one; or, as an educational experience, making us feel the suffering of others to appreciate the blessings of good health.

FINAL QUESTION AND ANSWERS

What determines the death of a human being according to Islamic law? Trustworthy doctors who believe in the sanctity of life can call for the stopping of medical support machines. The criterion should be whether or not the medical information reports, beyond doubt, death of both mind and heart. The death of only one does not allow the termination of life.

Can one choose to not be treated if medical treatment is possible? If medical treatment is available, then seeking medical support is required for patients and guardians.

What is the Islamic ruling on assisted suicide? Suicide is a major sin in Islam. One has to persevere in the face of sickness and ask God for support. God is the only one who has the right to end the life of a person.

CONCLUSION

Time has a beginning and an end. The human life has a beginning and an end; only God is before or after time. Actually, He is the creator of time and space. Collective time encompasses everything from the creation of the world to the passing of history, the warning of the impending judgment, the events of the day of resurrection, the final consignments, and passing into eternity. Everything that ever happened or ever may happen depends on God. All things surrender to God's will, even if unwillingly. Only human beings were given the choice to choose. Hence, we have been honored with the intuition to think and make decisions.

Yet, as we pass through this life, God expects us to live ethically and in accordance with God's divine rules known to us in the revealed scriptures. Maintaining God's creation with justice, equality, goodness, and peace is the least that is expected of all of us. We nurture life, as God wills, and we give God the right to take it away when He wills. Therefore, we are fully pleased with God's decrees and fully satisfied with His plans for us all.

Islamic faith is built in two basic messages: the oneness of God and the inevitability of the day of resurrection. Because God is one, human beings are enjoined to live lives of integrity and ethical and moral responsibility. God will render judgment on the quality of our ethical and moral lives. Therefore, life challenges are to be used to uplift us spiritually and morally. The way we carry out our lives and the way we die must be of a balanced nature, keeping in mind the need to live with dignity or die having preserved that dignity too. Those who are dying or those who help them die peacefully are, indeed, partners in the overall plan for how we stay in touch with God even as we prepare to transit to a new life.

Yahya Hendi is the Muslim chaplain at Georgetown University, the first American university to hire a full-time Muslim chaplain. He is also the Muslim chaplain at the National Naval Medical Center in Bethesda, Maryland. Imam Hendi is a Public Policy Conflict Resolution Fellow of the Center for Dispute Resolution of the University of Maryland School of Law and the Maryland Judiciary's Mediation and Conflict Resolution Office. He is the founder and president of Clergy beyond Borders and the founder and president of the new organization Imams for Universe, Dignity, Human Rights and Dialogue. He also serves as a member of the Islamic Jurisprudence Council of North America. He has served as an adjunct faculty member for Zanvyl Krieger School of Arts and Science and Osher's Lifelong Learning Institute of John Hopkins University; Fordham University; and Hartford Seminary. Imam Hendi also teaches a popular course at Georgetown University called Interreligious Encounter.

CHAPTER 14

Hindu Perspectives on End-of-Life Care

Suhita Chopra Chatterjee

The American melting pot has a large Hindu composition: approximately 1.5 million or 0.5% of the total population. It ranks among the world's top 10 countries with large Hindu populations. However, less than 0.5% were born in United States. Eighty-eight percent are of Asian origin.

Hindus in America are a highly cohesive group in terms of retaining their childhood members. More than eight in ten (84%) adults who were raised as Hindu still identify themselves as such. Age distribution of Hindus show that most are young: 58% are 30 to 49 years old and only 5% are over 65 years old. Hindus in the United States skew wealthier; in 2006, 43% had an annual pretax family income of $100,000 or more. (The Pew Forum on Religion and Public life, 2008)

HISTORY OF HINDUISM IN THE UNITED STATES

The history of U.S. Hinduism dates back to 1893 when Swami Vivekananda established the *Vedanta Society* based on a vision of the *Brahman* as the highest goal of life. Since then, several groups have been established in the United States. In 1920, Paramahansa Yogananda founded the Self-Realization Fellowship to disseminate his teachings on *Kriya Yoga*. In the late 1960s and 1970s, a number of gurus migrated and settled in the United States, bringing new streams of religious life. Maharishi Mahesh Yogi started the Students International Meditation Society (SIMS) in 1965. In the 1970s, Guru Maharaj-ji (the Divine Light Mission), Bhagwan Shree Rajneesh (Oshodhara), Swami Satchidananda (Integral Yoga International), Swami Rama (The Himalayan Institute), and Swami Muktananda (Siddha Yoga Dham movement) attracted visible followings and tried to bring East and West together in the practice of holistic health and yoga.

In the 1960s the *Bhakti* movement supplanted both the *Vedic* and the *Yogic* paths in the popular mind, and emphasized devotional love and service to Lord Krishna. Swami Bhaktivedanta Prabhupada built the first U.S. Krishna temple of the International Society for Krishna Consciousness (ISKCON).

There were also American-born seekers who themselves became Gurus in the 1970s, including Richard Alpert (who later became Ram Dass), Joyce Green (Ma Jaya Sati Bhagavati, spiritual teacher of Kashi Ashram), and Swami Chetanananda (Nityananda Institute) and drew on both Hindu and Buddhist dharma to articulate a teaching of service (see Pluralism Project).

Thus, we see that Hindus belong to various strands—Vedic, Bhakti, and the Yogic—representing the complex history of Hinduism in America. A break-up by different traditions shows that Vaishnavas constitute less than 0.3% of the total Hindu population; Shaivites, less than 0.3%; other Hindu groups, less than 0.3%; and those not specified, less than 0.3%. The Hindu American Foundation represents American Hindus and aims to educate people about Hinduism. Each group or movement established in America follows a particular *sampradaya,* or tradition handed down from the founder through successive religious teachers. Anand (2004) finds *particularity* as the essential feature of religious and group affiliation. She notes a boom in the formation and incorporation of Hindu religious organizations in the United States with over 500 organizations in the last two decades.

UNIFIED HINDU PHILOSOPHY OF DEATH: A MYTH OR A REALITY?

Given the fact that Hinduism in the United States represents a complex spiritual tradition, it is difficult to attribute a common philosophy of death. Unfortunately, service providers and planners have a tendency to homogenize reality and assume a unity in beliefs and values. Addressing the problem, Sarma (2005) feels that the desire to find a unifying and all-encompassing "essence" has constituted the greatest challenge to Hinduism among the diaspora in the United States.

Finding an essence is equally problematic in indigenous settings. Modernity and globalization have greatly transformed the religious world of Hindus. Considering that many U.S. Hindus are of Indian origin, a few observations pertaining to changes in death perspectives in India may throw light on the Hindu diaspora in America as well.

In India, orthodox Brahmanic Hinduism, associated most commonly with rituals, is undoubtedly on the wane and drastic changes are taking place in the way urban Hindus approach issues related to rites of passage. Complex ceremonies and rituals associated with death do not hold the same importance as they did for their ancestors and many funeral rites have been improvised.[1] For instance, *Jnana Probodhini*, a Pune-based organization, has cut short the period of defilement *(asudhi)* by devising a much shorter rite to be conducted in the home of the deceased over a 3-hour span—rites that normally extend until the 13th day after death. The introduction of electric crematoriums throughout India has also brought changes in cremation rituals and the symbolic representation of the corpse. While earlier, a flawless corpse on the pyre symbolized a flawless soul, today the removal of organs to benefit sick individuals has approval from community leaders and religious heads (Pandya, 2005).

Given the magnitude of changes in the Hindu way of death and dying, a coherent and "pure" Hindu perspective that influences end-of-life care among all the Hindus in America is difficult, if not largely erroneous. Indeed, Schombucher and Zoller's *Ways of Dying* shows the enormous variations that make it difficult to derive a universalistic model or theory of death in South Asia (1999). The best one can do is to generate an ideal type. One needs to bear in mind that age, education, income, caste, ties to ethnic community, place of immigration, affiliation to a particular sect, level of individual indoctrination to ideas, nature of disease, insurance provision, and social entitlement are all likely to impact attitudes toward death and dying. Again, grouping variables may generate spurious impressions. For instance, merely belonging to a particular sect does not signify much unless we know the level of indoctrination to the underlying philosophies and values. For instance, although most Hindus speak of detachment to the body, the mere fact of being a Hindu does not guarantee this unless one has practiced it as part of *sadhana* (religious practice). In other words, much finally depends on value-histories, patients' choices and preferences, family profile, and career needs. The best way, therefore, is to consult with the individual patient and family to explore individual needs or preference. Mitchell (2008) very rightly suggests that while manuals and guidelines on spiritual, religious, and cultural care are a guide, the only true approach is "to ask the person." In other words, we must

---

1 The rites related to the disposal of the dead are contained in the Vedic hymns. Some of these hymns were elucidated later in the *Brahmanas* and the *Aranyakas,* and then prescribed for religious usage through the *Grhya, Srauta* and *Asvalayana Sutras* (see Ghosh, 1989). A good exposition of the Hindu way of death is also provided by Rambachan Anantanaad, 2003.

avoid offering care in a stereotypical way while encouraging a distinct cultural passage to the finality of life.

DERIVING AN IDEAL TYPE: FURTHER CAUTIONARY NOTES

Service providers for Hindu communities in America need to take into account that while cultural sensitivity is an important tool for delivering the best outcomes, many sociopolitical and demographic factors are likely to impinge on patients' and families' attitudes toward the hospice approach to death and the services provided by such organizations. One cannot overlook the fact that the unique features of U.S. health delivery (e.g., its orientation toward technology and acute care) have given rise to concerns about costs, access, and quality even among American residents. Data suggest significant disparities in health status across racial, ethnic, socioeconomic groups, and between those who are insured and those who are not (Baldwin, 2003; Merrick, 2005). Under such circumstances, concerns are likely to be strongest among minority groups like the Hindus who, as the demographic data indicate, are highly educated and financially well off. It is probable that some of them may evince increased sensitivity to a program of care that does not provide aggressive technological intervention in life-prolongation. In other words, cultural sensitivity may at times appear to those who fear discrimination as a masking of more serious issues of justice and accountability.

The Hindu perspectives on end-of-life care contained in this chapter are based on metaphysical insights drawn from the *Bhagavad Gita* (the principal sacred text, irrespective of different strands of Hinduism in America), *Upanishads,* and the writings of modern exponents of Vedanta like Sri Aurobindo and Swami Abhedananda *Patanjali Yoga Sutra* (the *yogic* strands of Hindus draw their faith primarily from this text), and *Garuda Purana* (one of the *Vishnu Purunas,* it is considered highly ritualistic). These selectively focus on important beliefs, practices, and rituals that accompany the end of life and may provide help in developing critical sensitivities needed in caring for Hindu patients.

THE HINDU PHILOSOPHY OF DEATH

For want of a better expression, one may describe the Hindu philosophy as "death affirming." In the Bhagavad Gita, Lord Krishna's teachings on death posit four basic attitudes: the death of one's physical body is inevitable and should not cause prolonged grief; the subtle dimension of the person (*jiva*) does not die at death, but rather takes on a new body; the eternal Self (*atman*) is birthless and deathless and cannot be destroyed; and one who realizes the eternal Self while still alive will not be reborn but will merge with the ultimate reality, or Brahman.

According to Shri Aurobindo, there is a necessity and even justification of death, not as a denial, but as a process of life; death is necessary because eternal change of form is the sole immortality to which the finite living system can aspire, and eternal change of experience, the sole infinity to which the finite mind involved in living body can attain (ONLIFE, Online, n.d.).

Since death is inevitable, it should not cause fear; it is the *Mahaprasthana*—the great journey. When the lessons of life have been learned and when *karmas* reach intensity, the soul leaves the physical body, which then returns its elements to the earth. A devout Hindu therefore approaches death as a *sadhana* by bringing in a level of detachment. Any dread or anxiety itself is considered a result of an illusion that the unenlightened suffer from. The question "Who am I?" integrates the theme of death, what dies, and what is left out. In the highly imaginative confrontation of the ideal teacher (*Yama*, Lord of Death) with the student (named *Nachiketa*), it emerges that only deluded men identify with the body. Consequently, they consider death to occur when the body dies. The vulnerability to this belief itself leads to several lives and death. Strictly speaking, the Hindus want to escape not from *the* death, but from the jaws of several lives and deaths (see Katha Upanishad).

Death being the final journey, a "good death" is a voluntary renunciation of life and cremation is the sacrificial offering of the Self to the Gods. End-of-life care involves assisting the dying to conquer death by liberating oneself from the cycle of endless births. What are the best ways in which this can be done?

HOME AS THE PREFERRED LOCATION OF DYING

Many Hindus still believe that salvation is granted when one dies in a pilgrim place. However, since this is not always possible, the best option is to die at home where death can take place in *sumaran* (remembrance) of God and where deathbed rituals can be performed easily. According to Jindal (2008), many of the last wishes and desires of a patient may remain unfulfilled in a hospital. Therefore, healthcare teams need to accept this fact and comply with the request for home care.

Studies show that in the United States, very few terminally ill patients die at home. Pritchard's study of terminally ill patients at five teaching hospitals reveals that while 56% of patients died in acute care hospitals, only 25% died at home (See Merrick, 2005). Despite its low preference, home may perhaps be the best option for many Hindus. Since homecare is covered by Medicare and, in most cases, by Medicaid, doctors attending Hindu patients perhaps need to take homecare referrals more seriously.

VOLUNTARY RELINQUISHMENT OF LIFE

A controlled evacuation of the body is a sign of "good death" among Hindus. Death is a sacrificial offering of the self to God and the offering must be a complete act of renunciation with the help of a flawless body—an indicator of a flawless soul. It is for this reason that autopsies and organ donation are generally not acceptable. Long years of training in self-denial and meditation make it easy not only to deny life-prolonging treatment but also to forgo food and water, weakening the body such that the vital breath may leave it easily. Many elderly persons finding their duties adequately fulfilled and their body decaying with age and disease, prefer such active dying. Such deaths are indeed an occasion for celebration.[2] In fact, many Hindu monks have mastered the art of dying and an exemplary life invariably results in a "good death" (Swami Prabhananda, 2008). Counseling at the end of life for those who do not reach such spiritual heights involves assistance in calm acceptance of death. This may be the case for many who face uncontrolled and involuntary death—often designated as *akal mrityu* (untimely death) on account of disease, accident, and violence.

CONCENTRATING THE LIFE-ENERGY (*PRANA*): THE HALLMARK OF CONSCIOUS DYING

As indicated above, "good death" involves dying in a conscious state. Where the soul goes in the astral plane at death is dependent upon a person's earthly pursuits and the quality of the mind at death. The thoughts at death are the next *samskaras* (unconscious memories) of the astral body. Therefore, an important component of terminal care involves giving importance to the last moments of death and in performing the bedside rites according to scriptures. This has medically relevant consequences as far as administration of sense-deadening drugs or surgery is concerned for terminal patients. Following is an account of the rites for the righteous as illustrated in the Garuda Purana:

---

2 The willful cessation of life is carried to perfection in the practice of *Samadhi*, which results in conquest of the dualities of nature (love-hate, joy-sorrow) and also overcoming the will to live, which is considered as one of the hindrances to *Yoga* (Maharshi Patanjali, 1914).

The good person, finding his body, in its old age, afflicted with diseases, and the planetary conditions unfavorable, and not hearing the sounds of life,

And knowing his death to be near, should be fearless and alert, and should make reparation for any sins committed knowingly or in ignorance.

When it is near the time to die he must perform his ablutions, and worship Visnu in the form of Salagrama.

He must worship with fragrant substances, with flowers, with red saffron, with leaves of the holy basil, with incense, with lamps, with offerings of food and many sweetmeats, and other things.

He should give presents to Brahmins, should feed them with the offerings, and should recite the eight and the twelve syllabled mantras.

He should call to mind, and listen to, the names of Visnu and Siva. The name of Hari, coming with the range of hearing, takes away the sins of men.

Relatives, coming near the diseased, should not mourn. My holy name should be remembered and meditated upon repeatedly. (8:3–9)

He who calls, "O Ganges, Ganges" while life is flickering in the throat, goes when dead to the city of Visnu, and is not born again on earth.

And the man who, when his life is leaving, contemplates with faith the Ganges, goes to the highest goal.

Therefore he should contemplate, salute, keep in mind the Ganges, and drink its water. Then he should listen, however little, to the Bhagavata, which is a giver of liberation.

He who in his last moments repeats a verse, or half or quarter of a verse of the Bhagavata never returns hither from the world of Brahma.

The repeating of the Vedas and the Upanisads; the hymning of Visnu and Siva—these bring liberation at death to Brahmin Ksattriyas and Vasyas.

At the time when the breath is leaving the body, he should make a fast, O Bird. Dissatisfied with worldly things the twice-born should take up relinquishment.

He who says, while life is still flickering in his throat, "I have relinquished," goes at death to the city of Visnu, and is not born again on earth. (9:29–35)

CLEAR PROGNOSIS OF DEATH AS ASSISTANCE IN CONSCIOUS DYING

Conscious dying is possible when the prognosis of death is known to the patient. An important aspect of terminal care thus concerns the art of telling the truth and many Hindus prefer paternalistic decisions from the doctor. The dying may have both spiritual and material concerns. Hindu parents often have a strong desire that the children should share a common inheritance and mutual amity after their deaths. It is crucial that these concerns are properly and adequately addressed. A clear message from the doctor about the inevitability of death helps in finding timely solutions. False assurance of hope or wearing a mask of inaccessibility in front of the dying adult does not help. It only adds to the anxiety and depression with which the person already suffers (Jindal, 2008).

CONJOINING MEDICINE AND SPIRITUALITY: USE OF MULTIPLE THERAPEUTIC MODALITIES IN END-OF-LIFE CARE

Many Asian healing traditions conjoin medicine and spirituality in ways not yet adequately understood. For example, for many Hindu patients, the use of basil leaves for the dying is not merely a matter of ritual practice; it is deeply ingrained in the appreciation of the herb's medicinal properties.

Nursing professionals need to understand that culturally sensitive care might actually involve moving away from a biomedically centered scheme of caring to an integrated approach that allows multiple caring modules. Several therapeutic modalities may be used in end-of-life care, especially in pain management. When the biomedical model of treatment fails, many families may show noncompliance with its governed plans of action and resort to indigenous methods of healing and nutritional or dietary habits to comfort the patient, or even to counterbalance the disequilibrium caused by prolonged use of Western medicine. This is often disturbing for the service providers. For instance, in one survey of nurses from 67 hospices in the United States, the most common barriers to effective symptom management were identified as inability of family care providers to implement or maintain recommended treatments (38%) and patients and families not wanting recommended treatments (38%) (Johnson et al., 2005). Clearly, there is a need to outgrow this mind-set. There is always room for greater appreciation of the healing traditions and magico-religious rites of other cultures.

ENGAGING A DYING HINDU PATIENT: INTEGRATING SPIRITUAL DISCOURSES IN PALLIATIVE CARE

Hindu philosophy, as we have mentioned earlier, is death-affirming. Ideally, for the spiritually elevated, existential issues cease to have any relevance. In fact, spiritual elevation is defined in terms of one's ability to rise above existential angst. But not all patients reach such spiritual heights. Some may have intellectual understanding, but still feel unsure, left in a limbo, or not at peace.

The palliative care specialist's ability to positively intervene in the scene depends upon the sensitivity with which one can weave Hindu spiritual discourses in clinical practice or, in other words, integrate spirituality with medicine.

The major concerns of the dying and the corresponding spiritual interventions are presented below. The presentation is in the form of selective themes and issues rather than narratives. The actual adaptation of the themes needs to be made according to individual requirements. This exercise is meant for families and practitioners who feel that they don't know what to say or how to comfort the dying and the bereaved.

Death Anxiety

Patient: What is death? What happens to my body?

- Death is a process of life. The body dissolves and seeks new body forms in time to gain further experiences. The Soul, or *Atman*, never dies.
- "This is never born, nor does it die. It is not that, not having been, it again comes into being. This is unborn, eternal, changeless, ever-itself. It is not killed when the body is killed." (Swarupananda, 1909, 2:20)
- "As a person puts on new garments, giving up old ones, the soul similarly accepts new material bodies, giving up the old and useless ones." (2:22)
- "The wise soul is not born nor does it die.
  This one has not come from anywhere nor has it become anyone.
  Unborn, eternal, constant, primal,
  this one is not killed when the body is killed.
  If the killer thinks to kill,
  if the killed thinks oneself killed,
  both of these do not understand.
  This does not kill nor is it killed." — Katha Upanishad

Patient: Where will I go after death?

- "As are childhood, youth and old age, in this body, to the embodied soul, so also is the attaining of another body. Calm souls are not deluded thereat." (Swarupananda, 1909, 2:13)
- There is a distinction between gross and subtle body *(lingasarira)*, akin to the difference between outer and inner garment. The soul having enjoyed certain pleasures and having fulfilled certain desires leaves the gross body and manufactures another. The gross physical form of the body is one which has no existence and is constantly changing. It is not fixed or permanent which undergoes destruction with death. The lingasarira is the one which after cremation accompanies the transmigrating spirit. It is the essential link in the continuity of life because it is not destroyed by the death of the individual but continues to activate it throughout until it merges with the *Atman*, the True Self (Abhedananda, 1971).
- "The soul takes birth each time, and each time a mind, life and body are formed out of the materials of universal Nature according to the soul's past evolution and its need for the future. When the body is dissolved, the vital goes into the vital plane and remains there for a time, but after a time the vital sheath disappears. The last to dissolve is the mental sheath. Finally the soul or psychic being retires into the psychic world to rest there till a new birth is close." (Sri Aurobindo, quoted in ONLIFE Online, n.d.)

Family Concerns and Anxieties

Patient: All my dreams of having a happy family life are shattered.

- Look inwards. Focus on the process of creating your identity alone through nonattachment. All relationships are impermanent. Cultivate relationship with the permanent. Death may mean disconnection with friends and relatives, but it is also a time to reconnect with the Lord.

Anxiety Over Pain

Patient: The pain is unbearable. How will this pain end?

- Pain can be controlled through twofold processes. First, through the realization about the nature of pain, and second through the actual transcendence of it.
- "There is no distinction between pleasure and pain. All is, as it were, painful on account of everything bringing pain either as consequence or as anticipation of loss of happiness, or as fresh craving arising from impressions of happiness, and also as counteraction of qualities. We must

therefore learn to control all the dualities—good-bad, heat-cold and all the pains of opposites, including pain and pleasure." (Patanjali, 1914)

- "Pain and grief are Nature's reminder to the soul that the pleasure it enjoys is only a feeble hint of the real delight of existence. In each pain and torture of our being is the secret of a flame of rapture compared with which our greatest pleasures are only as dim flickerings. It is this secret which forms the attraction for the soul of the great ordeals, sufferings and fierce experiences of life which the nervous mind in us shuns and abhors." (ONLIFE, Online, n.d.)

Patient: And how do I control pain?

- The actual transcendence of all bodily processes including processes of pain start with yoga. "Yoga is concentration. It is the restrictions of the fluctuations of the mind stuff in which sources of all valid ideas are restricted. The calming of the affective states of mind takes place through different aids to yoga, regulation of breath and withdrawal of the sense organs. When there is restriction of the fluctuations (called *vriti)* of the mind stuff, there is concentration to an extent that there is no consciousness (of an object) including the body..." (Swami Vivekananda)
- One must not be moved by pain. Be calm. "That calm man who is same in pain and pleasure, whom these cannot disturb, alone is able, O great amongst men, to attain to immortality." (Swarupananda, 1909, 2:15)
- "How to avoid contact with the experience of pain? By understanding the structure of this experience. The division or the polarisation of experiencing into the experiencer and the experience, and the subsequent conjunction or contact of the subject and the object of the experiencing— and this can be avoided. Experiencing being the sole reality, the subject and the object are of identical nature, and thought is the dividing agent. Thought is of pain, pleasure, etc. and thought experiences pain, pleasure, etc., by the psychological action of division and contact. The possibility of the avoidance of pain is because of the unity of the seer (experiencer) and the seen (experience) without a division." (Patanjali, 1975, 2:17)

Patient: Will I unite with the Lord?

- "Controlling all the senses, confining the mind in the heart, drawing the *Prana* into the head, occupied in the practice of concentration, uttering the one-syllabled 'Om'—the Brahman, and meditating on Me—he who so departs, leaving the body, attains the Supreme Goal." (Swarupananda, 1909, 8:12–13)

Anxiety About Suffering

Patient: Why this suffering to me? I must have done evil in life to get this suffering.

- "Suffering is not inflicted as a punishment for sin or for hostility. Suffering comes like pleasure and good fortune as an inevitable part of life in ignorance. The dualities of pleasure and pain, joy and grief, good and ill fortune are the inevitable results of the ignorance which separates us from our true consciousness and from the divine." (ONLIFE, Online, n.d.)
- Life here is an evolution and the soul grows by experience, working out by it this or that in nature, and if there is suffering it is for the purpose of that working out, not a judgment inflicted by God or cosmic Law on the errors or stumbling which are inevitable in the ignorance.
- "Suffering has an important role to play. It is a necessary denial by the Divine. Only in an uplifting hour of stress men answer to the touch of greater things." (ONLIFE, Online, n.d.)

CREATING LIFE OUT OF DEATH: ASSISTING THE BEREAVED

Good end-of-life care involves helping the bereaved in many different ways which eventually lead to early resolution of grief. Hindu scriptures maintain that grief is a form of ignorance of the true facts of life and death. The funeral mantra says, "Grieve not for the ephemeral. [For] all this is but a form of life." According to Garuda Purana, "Relatives, coming near the diseased, should not mourn. My holy name should be remembered and meditated upon repeatedly." Gita also says, "Over the inevitable Thou shouldst not grieve" (2:27).

The Hindus dissociate as well as engage themselves with the dead. Death results in a polluting corpse on one hand and a malevolent ghost on the other hand. The first must be disposed of and the second must be transformed into a benevolent ancestor (*pitr*) through proper propitiatory rituals (Parry, 1994). Both require active help of community members.

Hinduism instructs cremation as soon as possible (unless the deceased is less than 3 years old). If the death takes place in a hospital or a hospice, a death certificate has to be arranged and the body has to be brought back home immediately, within 24 hours. It is then laid in the home's entryway on the floor and a lamp is lit up. At home, some may like to light a ritual fire (*homa*) with the help of a special funeral priest.

The body is washed and dressed by the relatives before taking it to the crematorium. Only men go to the crematorium, with the eldest son being the chief mourner. On returning home, after cremation, all bathe and share in cleaning the house and wear white clothes. A lamp is lit and a water pot is set where the body lay in state. A period of ritual impurity follows and the bereaved do not visit others' homes. But neighbors and relatives bring daily food to ease the burden of mourning. Twelve hours after cremation, family members return to collect the ashes in what is called the "bone gathering ceremony."

Post-cremation, *Sraddha* rites follow. The day after cremation, or 3, 10, or 13 days, depending on family traditions, the *sapindas* (those who have one or more ancestors in common going back to seven generations) perform *sraddha* rites on the river bank. Ritual feeding of rice balls (*Pindas*) symbolically ensures the formation of the subtle body and help it to adapt in a new condition. Finally, a feast is organized for the community members. These rituals are also repeated every year on the death anniversary (*Tithi*).

Providers need to be sensitive to the fact that the bereaved require help in performing the funeral rites according to customs. Although the Hindu community in the United States is fairly well knit, not all may have adequate networks and resources to meet with such exigencies. There might be families who require help washing and cremating the body and contacting the people of the community who may volunteer help. Some may show total unfamiliarity with American funeral homes and procedures for certifying death. A few may desperately wish to return to their homeland to dispose of their dead relatives but may find themselves stuck due to temporary visas and cumbersome immigration rules. Others may require help in arranging for the ashes to be sent back to their home town to be immersed in the holy waters.

Finally, there may be those left all alone without family support, facing intense loss with little opportunity for mourning due to work obligations. Such persons may need help moving on with life. Visiting the bereaved at home after death is not only comforting, but is considered a religious duty as well.

CONCLUSION

Ensuring a cultural passage to the final journey in life is a difficult task in a multicultural society. This chapter has highlighted select features for caregivers to remember when attending to Hindu patients and their families. Dying is an art among Hindus. But like all ancient art forms, only a few can appreciate it in modern times. Perhaps the real challenge lies in providing a facilitating environment that can remind the dying of their cultural roots even while in an alien environment—an environment where death is a matter of physiology and science and embroiled in issues of public policy and debates over rights and justice. Eventually, how Hindus die in the United States reveals much about how they live in a foreign land.

Suhita Chopra Chatterjee is presently working as a professor of sociology at the Department of Humanities and Social Sciences, Indian Institute of Technology, Kharagpur. Her current research areas include sociology of health and illness, medical sociology, and medical ethics. Her special interest is in the field of Death Studies.

References

Anand, P. (2004). Hindu diaspora and religious philanthropy in the United States. New York: Center on Philanthropy and Civil Society. Available at http://www.istr.org/conferences/toronto/workingpapers/anand.priya.pdf

Baldwin, D. M. (2003). Disparities in health and health care: Focusing efforts to eliminate unequal burdens. *Online Journal of Issues in Nursing, 8*(1).

Blank, R. H., & Merrick, J. C. (Eds.). (2005). *End-of-life decision making: A cross-national study.* Cambridge: MIT Press.

Chatterjee, S. C., Patnaik, P., & Chariar, V. M. (Eds.). (2008). *Discourses on aging and dying.* New Delhi: Sage.

Wood, E., & Subrahnabyam, S. V. (Trans.) (1911). *Garuda Purana.* Available at http://www.hinduwebsite.com/sacredscripts/puranas/gp/gp.asp

Ghosh, S. (1989). *Hindu concept of life and death.* Delhi: Munshiram Manoharlal.

Jindal, S. K. (2008). Old age, disease and terminal care: A Hindu perspective. In S. C. Chatterjee, P. Patnaik, & V. M. Chariar (Eds.), *Discourses on Aging and Dying* (pp. 217–224). New Delhi: Sage.

Johnson, D. C., Kassner, C. T., Houser, J., & Kutner, J. S. (2005). Barriers to effective symptom management in hospice. *Journal of Pain and Symptom Management, 29*(1), 69–79.

Beck, S. (Trans.) (1996). *Katha Upanishad.* Available at http://www.san.beck.org/Upan2-Katha.html

Kosmin, B. A., & Keysar, A. (2008). American Religious Identification Survey 2008. Available at http://www.americanreligionsurveyaris.org/reports/highlights.html

Melwani, L. (2007). Life and death in America: When Yama comes calling. Available at http://www.littleindia.com/news/135/ARTICLE/1895/2007-10-03.html

Merrick, J. C. (2005). Death and dying: The American experience. In R. H. Blank & J. C. Merrick (Eds.), *End-of-Life Decision Making: A Cross-national Study* (pp. 219–241). Cambridge, MA: MIT Press.

Mitchell, D. (2008). Spiritual and cultural issues at the end-of-life. *Palliative Care, 36*(2), 109–110.

Patanjali, M. (1975). *Enlightened living: A new interpretative translation of the Yoga Sutra of Maharsi Patanjali* (S. Venkatesananda, Trans.). The Chiltern Yoga Trust: Cape Town, South Africa. Available at http://www.swamivenkatesananda.org

Patanjali, M. (1914). *The yoga system of Patanjali* (J. H. Woods, Trans.). New Delhi: Motilal Banarsidass.

ONLIFE, Online. (n.d.). Question of the month. Available at http://www.sriaurobindosociety.org.in/qstarch/qstlist.htm

Pandya, S. K. (2005). End of life decision making in India. In R. H. Blank & J. C. Merrick (Eds.), *End-of-Life Decision Making. A Cross-national Study* (pp. 79–108). Cambridge: MIT Press.

Parry, J. P. (1994). *Death in Benaras.* New Delhi: Cambridge University Press.

Rambachan, A. (2003). The Hindu way of death. In C. D. Bryant (Ed.), *Handbook of Death and Dying* (2nd ed.), (pp. 640–648). Thousand Oaks, CA: Sage.

Sarma, D. (2005). The creation and transformation of Hinduism: A crisis of the holy. Papers presented by the Elijah Interfaith Academy Think Tank in preparation for the second meeting of World Religious Leaders.. Available at http://www.elijah-interfaith.org/materials/conference-proceedings/crisis-of-the-holy.html

Schombucher, E., & Zoller, C. P. (Eds). (1999). *Ways of dying: death and its meaning in South Asia.* New Delhi: Manohar.

Swarupanada, S. (1909). *Srimad Bhagavad Gita*. Calcutta: Advaita Ashrama.

Abhedananda, S. (1971). *Life beyond death*. Kolkata: Ramakrishna Vedanta Math.

Prabhananda, S. (2008). The art of dying with dignity. In C. S. Chatterjee, P. Patnaik, & V. M. Chariar, (Eds.), *Discourses on Aging and Dying* (pp. 60–82). New Delhi: Sage.

Vivekananda, S. (2004). *Raja Yoga or conquering the eternal nature*. Kolkata: Advaita Ashrama.

The Pew Forum on Religion and Public Life. (2008). U.S. religious landscape survey. Available at http://religions.pewforum.org/

The Pluralism Project. (n. d.) The rush of the gurus. Available at http://pluralism.org/ocg/CDROM_files/hinduism/rush_of_gurus.php

CHAPTER 15

Buddhist Perspectives on End-of-Life Care

Betty J. Kramer

Faced with a fairly fragmented healthcare system of specialists that views death as the enemy, places emphasis on care and treatment of the physical body, is aversive to acknowledging suffering, and is driven by medical technology to prevent death at all costs (Callahan, 2003; Gordon, Blackhall, Bastis, & Thurman, 2002), U.S. medical professionals are inadequately prepared to address spiritual needs and alleviate suffering at the end of life. Medical students in the United States report substantially less training and preparedness in palliative and end-of-life care than even their British counterparts (Hammel, Sullivan, Block, & Twycross, 2007). In striking contrast, many Eastern cultures, grounded in Buddhist philosophy and teachings, have spent centuries developing the science of mind and spirit, placing emphasis on understanding nonphysical dimensions of health and spiritual well-being and development. Buddhist philosophy promotes deeply embracing the inescapable truth of impermanence (i.e., the inevitability of death), the interdependence of existence, the truth of suffering, and developing compassion for all living beings. From these teachings and practices handed down through the centuries has come a sophisticated understanding of the subtle stages of the dying process and what care providers can and should do to promote the most optimal outcome for the dying individual (Sogyal Rinpoche, 1994). Thus, Buddhist philosophy, psychology, and teachings about death and dying offer valuable perspectives and practical instructions for professional caregivers (Gordon, Blackhall, Bastis, & Thurman, 2002; Coberly, 2002).

In addition to what hospice and palliative care professionals may personally gain from Buddhist wisdom, understanding foundational Buddhist beliefs, practices, and rituals is necessary to more competently meet the needs of the dramatically growing number of U.S. Buddhists and those who hold Buddhist beliefs who will require care at the end of their lives. Evidence from two recent national surveys conducted by the Pew Research Center, an independent opinion research group, reported that the religious landscape in the United States is changing rapidly. Twenty-eight percent of Americans have left the faith in which they were raised, 75% of U.S. Buddhists have converted to Buddhism, and nearly one-quarter of the population has adopted foundational beliefs associated with Eastern religions (Pew Forum, 2010a, 2010b). There has been a 170% growth in Buddhist affiliation from 1990 to 2001 alone (Sensei, 2010). The purpose of this chapter is to offer a historical perspective of Buddhism in America; describe foundational Buddhist beliefs, practices, and rituals associated with death and dying; highlight practical advice for professionals caring for Buddhists; and describe Buddhist hospice and training programs and online resources.

HISTORICAL PERSPECTIVE ON BUDDHISM IN AMERICA

Buddhism, the fourth largest religion in the world, is the fastest growing religion in the United States (Morgan, 2004). The origin of Buddhism can be traced from India, where the Hindu Prince Siddhartha, deeply troubled by the suffering in the world, left his life of luxury at the age of 29 to seek understanding of the deeper meaning of life and how to end suffering. After abandoning 6 years of extreme austerity practices, he realized that pain and starvation would not help him realize Enlightenment. He accepted sweet milk and a meal of rice, left the other ascetics he had practiced with, and resolved to sit in meditation under a papal tree until he found Enlightenment (Seager, 1999). Throughout the night in a deep state of mental absorption, he experienced the most profound awakening as he:

> observed the unfolding of his own many past lives...saw how karma influenced the shaping of events both in the present moment and in the future...analyzed how karma worked to trap human beings in samsara, and he discovered a path or method to follow to gain liberation, an experience generally referred to as *nirvana*. (Seager, 1999, p. 13)

He became known as the *Buddha*, meaning the *awakened* or *enlightened* one. For the next 45 years, he traveled extensively giving teachings, referred to as *the dharma* (the doctrine), sharing his profound insights that led many others to the awakened state. Considered the foundation of his teachings, the Four Noble Truths highlight the truth and nature of suffering of all living beings, the truth regarding the causes of suffering, the truth that suffering can cease, and the truth of the noble Eightfold Path for how to end suffering and attain awakening (i.e., Morgan, 2004; Seager, 1999).

Some time after his death, the dharma followed two paths as it spread to the rest of Asia (Landaw & Bodian, 2003), disseminating two main branches in Buddhism known as *Theravada* and *Mahayana* (Seager, 1999). Theravada Buddhism spread to Sri Lanka, Burma, Thailand, Laos, and Cambodia. The Theravada, considered the most orthodox branch, is deeply rooted in the monastic tradition and places emphasis on ethical integrity by following the Five Precepts (i.e., no killing, stealing, lying, sexual misconduct, and intoxicants), engaging in virtuous actions, and practicing meditation to achieve *samatha* (i.e., tranquility achieved through concentration on an object) and *vipassana* (i.e., insight) (Morgan, 2004). The tradition of Mahayana Buddhism spread to China, Korea, Japan, Vietnam, Tibet, and Mongolia (Landaw & Bodian, 2003). A distinguishing feature in the Mahayana is the ideal of the *Bodhisattva*, one who takes vows to dedicate their life to attaining enlightenment so that they may then work to free all other sentient beings from *samsara* (i.e., cyclic existence of birth, death, and rebirth). Opened more broadly to lay persons and the ordained, individuals following this tradition practice the six perfections in daily life (i.e., patience, generosity, ethics, joyous effort, concentration, and wisdom), and through meditation seek to develop altruistic great compassion and transcendent wisdom (i.e., to understand the nature of reality of inherent emptiness and dependent origination). An extension of the Mahayana is the *Vajrayana* or the "Diamond Vehicle" that was most completely developed in Tibet and surrounding regions of central Asia (Seager, 1999). This path, considered "the swift path" because it is possible to attain complete enlightenment in one lifetime, requires the guidance of a well-qualified, realized teacher who offers individual instruction suited to the needs of the student, transmits and disseminates the dharma, and instructs the student in purification practices, mind training, and the transformative meditation practices (Morgan). There are four schools of Tibetan Buddhism, each with its own lineage and distinctive traditions and practices.

During the 19th century, Buddhist thought arrived in the United States through the transcendentalist and theosophy movement and writers such as Walt Whitman, Henry David Thoreau, and Ralph Waldo Emerson (Seager, 1999). Intrigued with the religions of Asia, these individuals inspired future generations of poets and writers of the Beat generation such as Allen Ginsberg, Gary Snyder, and Jack Kerouac, who helped popularize Zen Buddhism during the 1950s and 1960s. In the 1970s, American travelers to Southeast Asia including Jack Kornfield, Sharon Salzburg, and Joseph Goldstein, who studied with masters in the Theravada tradition, returned to co-found the Insight Meditation Society in Barer, Massachusetts in 1975 that precipitated the dramatic growth of vipassana and insight meditation practice in the United States (Landaw & Bodian, 2003). The invasion of Tibet in the 1950s by the communist Chinese government brought many Tibetan lamas and the Vajrayana to the United States. As will be described below, many of these teachers have made important contributions to our understanding of the death and dying process and how to care for the dying more skillfully. "Engaged Buddhism," first introduced in the 1960s by Thich Nhat Hanh, has drawn many American followers to the study and application of mindfulness and Buddhist thought to the social problems of modern life. Changes in immigration law in 1965 also substantially contributed to the growth of Buddhism in the United States (Seager, 1999). Although Zen, Tibetan, and Vipassana have most profoundly influenced Western culture and are prominent forms of U.S. Buddhism today, the Buddhist spiritual landscape remains extremely diverse, including 13% of U.S. Buddhists who choose not to affiliate with any of the traditions (Morgan, 2004). One national survey investigating organizational level data on 231 Buddhist centers in the United States reported that current organizations practice one or more of 31 different forms of Buddhism, originating from 27 countries (Smith, 2007). With a low response rate of 23%, the diversity is likely much greater.

Foundational Beliefs

There are several foundational and pervasive Buddhist beliefs useful for healthcare providers to understand for providing culturally and spiritually competent care.

Truth of Impermanence: Preliminary practices in Buddhism encourage individuals to deeply contemplate impermanence and the precious nature of a human life in order to inspire sincere effort in spiritual practice. Guided meditations and contemplations offered by Western Buddhist teachers and writers facilitate heightened awareness and understanding of this truth that may be a useful antidote for healthcare professionals steeped in a death-denying culture (Halifax, 2008; Levine, 1997).

Reincarnation: Rather than viewing life as beginning with birth and ending with death, the Buddhist view holds that life is just one of a series of lives. The essence mind—a formless mind continuum—departs from the body and takes rebirth into a new life form (Sogyal Rinpoche, 1994). Rebirth may occur from a few moments to several weeks following death, and this cycle of birth, life, death, and rebirth will continue over innumerable lifetimes until one has purified all of one's negative actions and achieved enlightenment.

Karma: Karma is the law of cause and effect. It simply means that all actions of body, speech, and mind, will leave subtle imprints on the mind that will remain until they ripen in current or future lives as happiness or suffering, depending on whether actions are virtuous or nonvirtuous, or until they are cleansed or purified by spiritual practices (Morgan, 2004).

Potential for Awakening: At the very "heart of the Buddha's teaching lies the idea that the potential for awakening and perfection is present in every human being and that it is a matter of personal effort to realize that potential" (Dalai Lama, quoted in Goldstein, 2002, p. ix). The teachings of the Buddha, referred to as the dharma, offer clear sequential methods for awakening that include actions to both avoid and to cultivate. Although the emphasis placed on different methods for awakening varies by tradition, enlightenment becomes possible by avoiding harmful actions of body, speech, and mind; taming and developing a calm and focused mind; developing wisdom and altruistic great compassion; and engaging in actions to benefit others and to perfect virtuous qualities. "In some Buddhist traditions, notably the Tibetan, it is believed that advanced practitioners can use the time after death to develop greater meditative absorption" and achieve enlightenment via the dying process (Cousens, 2004, p. 4). Training the mind and preparing for death through lifelong meditation practices are central to Vajrayana practice.

The Death Process: In contrast to the Western belief that death occurs the moment brain activity ceases, the Buddhist view is that the death process is complete when the essence-mind exits the body, which may be up to 3 days after the cessation of vital signs that represent just one of the stages of the death process (Coberly, 2002). According to the Tibetan Buddhist teachings,

> The individual who is in the process of passing away is energetically returning to their source, literally reabsorbed into his or her original being. This process can go on for a significant amount of time before that individual passes away. And during that time the individual needs a very different kind of care, in order for that process to go smoothly. (Domo Geshe Rinpoche, as cited in Grand Transitions Institute, 2010).

There are eight stages of the dying process. Each of these stages coincide with the dissolution of energies related to the five elements (earth, water, fire, wind, and space) and the aggregates of individuality such as forms, feelings, discriminations, compositional factors, and ordinary consciousness (Coberly, 2002). Although a full description of this dissolution process is beyond the scope of this chapter, hospice care professionals may find it helpful to be familiar with the external signs of these stages and the implications for providing end-of-life care at each of these stages (see chart created by Coberly, 2002, pp. 94–98). Some of the signs that the consciousness has left the body include: absence of heat of the heart, smell emanating from the body, the skin failing to return to its proper place when pressed, or a trickle of fluid coming from the nostrils (Lama Zopa Rinpoche, 2008a).

State of Mind at the Time of Death: A foundational Buddhist belief that has profound implications for care providers is that the actual dying experience and one's state of mind at the time of death will profoundly influence the quality of one's next rebirth. *Liberation in the Palm of your Hand* (Pabongka Rinpoche & Trijang Rinpoche, 2006), details the steps on the path to enlightenment as presented in a 24-day teaching given by the great Tibetan lama Kyabje Pabongka Rinpoche near Lasa in 1921 to a group of 700 monks, nuns, and lay people. According to this classic spiritual text, "Your dying thoughts activate the karma that will throw you into the next rebirth after that death. ...If your dying thoughts are of faith, and so on (compassion)...your virtue will be activated. It is therefore vital to pray with virtuous thoughts...while mind is still active and still has course form of recognition" (Pabongka Rinpoche & Trijang Rinpoche, 2006, pp. 476–477). His Holiness the Dalai Lama has said "at the moment of death...if we make special effort to generate a virtuous state of mind, we may strengthen and activate a virtuous karma, and so bring about a happy rebirth (Sogyal Rinpoche, 1994, p. ix).

PRACTICES AND RITUALS

Common practices and rituals across traditions performed by Buddhists in daily life include taking refuge, making offerings, and engaging in some form of meditation. Taking refuge is a daily vow, often repeated three times, in which the individual vows to turn to the Buddha, the dharma, and the sangha as a "source of spiritual guidance and support" (Landaw & Bodian, 2003, p. 133). Buddhists typically create a small altar in their homes where they have sacred images and make offerings that serve as a sacred focal point for meditation. At the end of life, Buddhists may want to have a small altar and sacred images in their visual field to continue these important rituals.

The practices and rituals associated specifically with dying vary across the different traditions. For example, prayers and meditation practices that may be encouraged during or after the dying process as well as the duration of time they may be carried out are influenced by culture and tradition. Lama Zopa Rinpoche of the Gelugpa lineage in the Tibetan Buddhist tradition emphasizes two main practices for the time of death: the *Medicine Buddha Puja* and the *Eight Prayers for the Time of Death*. He offers several additional mantras and prayers that may be practiced to benefit the deceased (2008b). Pragmatic considerations such as how the body should be handled or treated after death, the length of time that a body should be left undisturbed, and whether the body is buried or cremated will vary if one is a Western, Tibetan, Japanese, Korean, or Taiwanese Buddhist. Results from an Australian survey of Buddhists from the Theravada and Mahayana traditions and different countries of origin illustrate some variability in customary practices during the dying process, at the time of death, and after death (Cousens, 2004). End-of-life ritual prayers for Tibetan Buddhists and implications for spiritual and religious assessment—including the Phowa death preparation ritual practiced by some in this tradition—are described by Smith-Stoner (2006), although these, too, will vary depending upon the particular school of Tibetan Buddhism.

PRACTICAL ADVICE FOR PROFESSIONALS CARING FOR BUDDHIST PATIENTS

Given the diversity in countries of origin and types and forms of Buddhism practiced in the United States today, as well as the tremendous variability in the practices and rituals across traditions, care providers will need to individually determine what is customary according to the beliefs, practices, culture, and tradition of the individual they are caring for. Thus, the most important advice is to listen deeply to ascertain the individual's wishes and preferences and to determine the origin and form of their Buddhist beliefs and practices. If they have a guru or lama, it will be especially important to consult with these spiritual authorities for their instruction regarding the most appropriate care and practices related to the dying process. For those who belong to a Buddhist spiritual community, monks, nuns, or lay practitioners could offer valuable expertise and will likely want to be involved in providing care, support, and reciting special prayers and mantras (Rapgay, 2006).

Most of what has been published concerning Buddhist perspectives and practical advice for caring for the dying has been written by Tibetan Buddhist masters or seasoned practitioners. As such, the practical advice put forth in this chapter is drawn from this tradition. Some of these publications are specifically for Tibetan Buddhist students and those who care for them at the end of life (see text and audio course by Lama Zopa Rinpoche, 2008a), but the majority of publications provide pragmatic guidance for compassionate care for the dying regardless of religious orientation (Bokar Rinpoche, 1993; Hookham, 2006; Rapgay, 2006; Sogyal Rinpoche, 1994). One of the most influential books is the international bestseller *The Tibetan Book of the Living and Dying* (Sogyal Rinpoche, 1994), which offers inspiring perspectives on the meaning of life, how to accept death, how to care for the dying, and what happens during and following the death process. In a general sense, and consistent with preferences across the traditions, what is most emphasized is the importance of providing a suitable atmosphere for the person to die peacefully and to help the person die with a calm, peaceful, and uplifted mind (Kongsuwan & Touhy, 2009). This important point and other practical instructions across the dying trajectory are described below.

In the Weeks Prior to Death: Primary suggestions for the weeks prior to death include trusting the patient to dictate how much pain medication they need while avoiding unnecessary sedation, listening deeply to engage the patient in discussions about what they wish to discuss rather than pushing one's own agenda, expressing and offering forgiveness (if relevant), encouraging the patient to express positive emotions such as love and kindness to others, and encouraging reflection upon and rejoicing in the virtuous activities they have engaged in (Chodron, 2010; Khadro, 2010). Individuals who experience regrets from their past actions may benefit from requesting forgiveness, making amends, or making confessions to one's spiritual teacher or other sources of refuge (Cousens, 2004). Buddhist practitioners may wish to have a small altar in their immediate environment that would include spiritual objects to support their practice such as an image of their teacher or the Buddha, offerings, and their prayer beads (i.e., a *mala*). It is important to Buddhist practitioners to enhance their faith, devotion, and confidence in their practice, personal deities, spiritual teachers, and other objects of refuge. To uplift the minds of Buddhist patients, family members and caregivers may share inspiring, uplifting stories and encourage altruistic great compassion and aspiration to continue one's spiritual practice through death, the intermediate state, and future lives (Khadro, 2010). To relinquish attachments, practice generosity, and feel greater peace of mind, many Buddhists (and non-Buddhists) may find it helpful to organize their will and disperse their possessions well prior to their death (Cousens, 2004).

Just Preceding the Time of Death or During the Active Dying Process: Suggestions include maintaining a peaceful and calm environment—avoiding strong clinging, displays of emotion, or actions and discussions that may be distressing to the patient (e.g., sobbing, shouting, criticizing, or getting angry); using the language of their own faith to encourage them to arise loving thoughts toward others and to have faith; saying prayers or reciting mantra silently or aloud as they are dying; and supporting and trusting the patient in their individual dying process (Chodron, 2010). This would include creating a serene and uplifting environment with lovely views, flowers, pictures, or images of holy beings as well as the removal or avoidance of objects, experiences, or interactions that might generate strong attachment, fear, anxiety, or anger. Interventions should ameliorate anxiety and other troubled states of mind and help the person feel safe, relaxed, and at ease. For example, if the patient doesn't like a caregiver, they may develop angry or agitated thoughts that will create more negative states of mind. Alternating caregivers, helping caregivers better address patient concerns, or helping the patient explore more positive ways of viewing the situation may be necessary. The person may be encouraged to reflect on the virtues of holy or enlightened beings (Cousens, 2004). Family members may wish to assure the individual that they will take care of anything that is of concern and they themselves will be fine following the death (Cousens, 2004). Well-trained Buddhists will not cry or express strong emotion during the dying process (Khadro, 2010). A private space away from the body for family members or friends who experience strong emotions should be available. As the dissolution process advances and the individual is no longer responsive to the outer environment, it is preferable to avoid touching, massaging, or moving the body. In the Tibetan Buddhist tradition, it is believed that directing the consciousness through touch or sound to lower parts of the individual's body or parts other than the crown of their head may "draw them into a less than favourable rebirth" (Hookham, 2006, p. 140).

Following the Death: It is suggested to leave the body untouched for 3 days or as long as possible unless signs that the consciousness has left the body are present (Chodron, 2010). The first touch to the body should be to the crown of the head while one whispers a directive for them to "Go to heaven or to a safe place," "Go to the pure land," or "Take a precious human rebirth," depending upon their belief system (Chodron, 2010). According to Buddhist teachings, following death—when one's consciousness is in the intermediate state before rebirth—they may float freely and be highly receptive to the thoughts of others (Hookham, 2006). Thus, maintaining compassionate and virtuous thoughts about the deceased is advised. Another important suggestion is to dedicate and to express in thought or words your wishes for their peaceful transition and for an optimum human rebirth. Donations to charities in the name of the deceased are often appreciated by Buddhists and may be encouraged by the family because they are seen to collect merit for the dead (Cousens, 2004). Post-death rituals should be followed according to one's tradition and culture.

BUDDHIST HOSPICE AND TRAINING PROGRAMS IN THE UNITED STATES

Several U.S. Buddhist organizations have been influential in transforming the culture of living and dying to be more mindful and compassionate and better meet the spiritual, physical, and emotional needs of the dying regardless of one's religious or spiritual orientation. These include Buddhist hospice programs such as the Zen Hospice Project (2010) founded in 1987; spiritual care respite, Buddhist chaplaincy, and end-of-life care training programs such as those offered by the New York Zen Center for Contemplative Care (2010); and other prominent spiritual care training programs for hospice volunteers and professionals such as the *Spiritual Care Education and Training Program* offered by the Rigpa Fellowship (2010), the year-long *End-of-Life Care Practitioner Program* offered by the Metta foundation (2010), and the Upaya Zen Center's (2010) *Project on Being with Dying,* developed by Roshi Joan Halifax. Another training program is offered as part of the Grand Transitions Institute (2010) that has recently started a volunteer-based and donation-funded Buddhist hospice and currently offers a *Conscious End-of-Life Training Program* to prepare professionals and volunteers who want to prepare for their own eventual dying process and gain the skills to provide a careful, energetic spiritual care environment for those who are actively dying. Tara Home (2010), affiliated with Land of Medicine Buddha in California, is a home for terminally ill individuals enrolled in a hospice program who simultaneously receive care by Tara Home's family of volunteers trained to provide support services and meet emotional and spiritual needs in partnership with the hospice staff.

CONCLUSION

In summary, many Buddhists practice for death over the course of their life, seeking to cultivate virtuous states of mind and abandon harmful and suffering states of mind so they may have no regrets and be better prepared to hold a virtuous state of mind at the time of death. Buddhists deliberately cultivate awareness of the certainty of death, the preciousness of life, and the uncertainty of the timing of death to support their commitments to make spiritual progress. Although there are some commonalities in foundational beliefs in the teachings of the Buddha and in some of the practices and rituals, there is tremendous variability and diversity that professionals must understand in working with Buddhist patients. While practical wisdom from the Tibetan Buddhist tradition offers pragmatic instructions for compassionate care for the dying, individual assessments tailored to the distinctive needs, beliefs, and values of the individual are essential to culturally and spiritually competent care of Buddhists in America.

Betty J. Kramer, PhD, MSSW, is a professor in the School of Social Work and a member of the Comprehensive Cancer Center at the University of Wisconsin-Madison. With her colleagues, she established competencies and a national research agenda for social work research in palliative and end-of-life care. With support from the John A. Hartford and the Open Society Institute and Soros Foundation, Dr. Kramer has implemented several projects relevant to improving care of the dying. She is a faculty member and mentor of a National Cancer Institute training grant. As a Fellow of the Center for Contemplative Mind in Society, Dr. Kramer is developing curriculum focusing on the importance of mindfulness and the use of meditation as a therapeutic intervention. She has 28 years' experience with various forms of meditation, a longstanding interest in Eastern perspectives on mental health, and is a practitioner of Tibetan Buddhism. Recent awards include the Association for Gerontology Education in Social Work (AGE-SW) Faculty Achievement Award (2004) and the National Hospice and Palliative Care Organization (NHPCO) Distinguished Researcher Award (2008).

REFERENCES

Bokar Ripoche (1993). *Death and the art of dying in Tibetan Buddhism.* San Francisco: ClearPoint Press.

Callahan, D. (2003). Living and dying with medical technology. *Critical Care Medicine, 31*(5 Suppl.), S344–S346.

Chodron, T. (2010). *Venerable Thubton Chodron's home page: Death and dying: Preparing for a loved one's death.* Retrieved September 3, 2010 from http://www.thubtenchodron.org/DeathAndDying/preparing_for_a_loved_ones_death.html

Coberly, M. (2002). *Sacred passage: How to provide fearless, compassionate care for the dying.* Boston: Shambala Publications.

Cousens, D. (2004). *Buddhist care for the dying.* Footscray West, Victoria: Buddhist Council of Victoria.

Goldstein, J. (2002). *One Dharma: The emerging western Buddhism.* San Francisco: Harper Collins.

Gordon, J. S., Blackhall, L., Bastis, M. K., & Thurman, R. A. F. (2002). Asian spiritual traditions and their usefulness to practitioners and patients facing life and death. *Journal of Alternative and Complementary Medicine, 8,* 603–608.

Grand Transitions Institute (2010). *For a conscious end of life.* Available from http://www.grandtransitions.org

Halifax, R. J. (2008). *Being with dying: Cultivating compassion and fearlessness in the presence of death.* Boston: Shambhala.

Hammel, J. F., Sullivan, A. M., Block, S., & Twycross, R. (2007). End-of-life and palliative care education for final-year medical students: A comparison of Britain and the United States. *Journal of Palliative Medicine, 6,* 1356–1366.

Hookham, S. (2006). *There's more to dying than death: A Buddhist perspective.* Birmingham, UK: Windhorse Publications.

Khadro, S. (2010). *A Buddhist's death.* Retrieved September 2, 2010, from http://www.amitabhahospice.org/public/helpful_info/buddhist_death.php

Kongsuwan, W., & Touhy, T. (2009). Promoting peaceful death for Thai Buddhists: Implications of holistic end-of-life care. *Holistic Nursing Practice, 23,* 289–296.

Levine, S. (1997). *A year to live: How to live this year as if it were your last.* New York: Bell Tower.

Lama Zopa Rinpoche. (2008a). *Heart advice for death and dying.* Portland, OR: FPMT Education Publications.

Lama Zopa Rinpoche. (2008b). *Heart practices for death and dying.* Portland, OR: FPMT Education Publications.

Landaw, J., & Bodian, S. (2003). *Buddhism for dummies.* Hoboken, NJ: Wiley Publishing, Inc.

Metta Foundation. (2010). *End-of-life care practitioner course.* Available from http://www.mettainstitute.org/EOLprogram.html

Morgan, D. (2004). *The Buddhist experience in America.* Westport, CT: Greenwood Press.

New York Zen Center for Contemplative Care. (2010). *New York Zen center for contemplative care.* Available from http://www.zencare.org/index.html

Pabongka Rinpoche & Trijang Rinpoches (2006). *Liberation in the palm of your hand: A concise discourse on the path to enlightenment.* Boston: Wisdom Publications.

Pew Forum. (2010a). *U.S. religious landscape survey.* Available from http://religions.pewforum.org/pdf/report-religious-landscape-study-key-findings.pdf

Pew Forum. (2010b). *Many Americans mix multiple faiths: Eastern, New Age beliefs widespread.* Accessed September 1, 2010, from http://pewforum.org/Other-Beliefs-and-Practices/Many-Americans-Mix-Multiple-Faiths.aspx

Rapgay, L. (2006). A Buddhist approach to end-of-life care. In C. M. Puchalski (Ed.), *A time for listening and caring: Spirituality and the care of the chronically ill and dying* (pp. 131–137). New York: Oxford University Press.

Rigpa. (2010). *Rigpa: Spiritual care education and training programme.* Available from http://www.rigpa.org

Seager, R. H. (1999). *Buddhism in America.* New York: Columbia University Press.

Sensei, S. (2010). *Buddhism in America.* Available from http://buddhistfaith.tripod.com/pureland_sangha/id65.html

Smith, B. G. (2007). Research note: Variety in the Sangha: A survey of Buddhist organizations in America. *Review of Religious Research, 48,* 308–317.

Smith-Stoner, M. (2006). Phowa: End-of-life ritual prayers for Tibetan Buddhists. *Journal of Hospice and Palliative Nursing, 8,* 357–363.

Sogyal Rinpoche (1994). *The Tibetan Book of living and dying.* San Francisco: HarperCollins.

Tara Home. (2010). *Tara Home: Compassionate care for the end of life.* Available from http://tarahome.org

Upaya Zen Center. (2010). *Being with dying: Professional training programs in contemplative end-of-life care.* Available from http://www.upaya.org/bwd

Zen Hospice Project. (2010). *What we do.* Available from http://www.zenhospice.org/prod

CHAPTER 16

Spiritual Care for Agnostics and Atheists at the End of Life

Marilyn Smith-Stoner

Life is a banquet, but at some point, even at great banquet,
you get tired.

You look around and say, "How do I get out of here?"

This chapter is about nonbelievers—about people who do not believe in life after death, divine intervention, or a god of any kind. This community of nonbelievers goes by many names, including atheists, skeptics, and humanists. Much of the information included here comes from my years of experience collaborating with nonbelievers. Where there is research, I have included it. However, there is a dearth of formal research-based studies. Therefore, the evidence presented is derived from experts in the field, my extensive communication with this community, and a review of printed material. Atheist colleagues have reviewed this chapter and commented on it prior to publication.

MY INTEREST IN ATHEISTS

After successfully publishing articles on Tibetan Buddhist issues related to end-of-life care, I wanted to deepen my own understanding of other diverse groups of people, especially those that are not well understood by members of the hospice profession. My immediate choice was to study atheists since I had observed numerous problems with patients and staff members related to unwanted preaching about God and salvation over the years.

Since the publication of my preliminary study of *End-of-Life Preferences for Atheists*, and the referencing of this article by Richard Dawkins, noted British atheist, I have been in regular discussion with atheists throughout the world. During the last year or so, I have worked extensively in large healthcare organizations in California and continue to find conflict among staff and patients who are nonbelievers. Staff members, especially, object to being continually exposed to religious rituals in the workplace. Their concerns will also be discussed at the end of the chapter. My hope is that readers will be able to use the information to honor the nonbelief of millions of potential hospice patients, their family members, and colleagues.

An important assumption of this chapter is that the group of people collectively known as *atheists* is composed of loving, caring, ethical members of society who actively work for the betterment of humanity. Like other members of society, they are complete, fully functioning people without a belief in any religious dogma. If one is referring to their sense of meaning in life, to their love of friends and family, and their desire to enjoy and preserve the earth, then they are all spiritual. A study participant described a common worldview: "I simply believe that we are born, live, and die in a largely random manner in which we have limited opportunities, and no supernatural entities control our destiny" (Smith-Stoner, 2007).

Beyond this general view is a wide range of perspectives. No patients or family members with this worldview need to be saved from, or by, the hospice team.

WHO IS AN ATHEIST?

The estimates of the number of atheists vary worldwide. At the very least, there are millions. The various labels or descriptors used to describe this philosophy also complicates the issues. Terms include agnostics, atheists, nonbelievers, skeptics, humanists, unbelievers, nonreligious, and many others. As with any community, there are a variety of descriptors and beliefs within each of the descriptors.

Like most groups, individuals who do not believe in a god or afterlife have a broad range of beliefs and labels to describe themselves. Here are a few of the more common labels with their definitions:

1. *Atheist:* a person who does not believe in the existence of God or gods (Oxford Dictionary, 2010).
2. *Agnostic:* a person who believes that nothing is known or can be known of the existence or nature of God (Oxford Dictionary, 2010).
3. *Humanist:* Good without God, a belief in life before death (Epstein, 2009).
4. *Skeptic:* a person inclined to question or doubt accepted opinions. Also a person who doubts the truth of Christianity and other religions; an Atheist (Oxford Dictionary, 2010).

The term *atheist* will be used to refer to this group of individuals.

The spiritual definition adopted for palliative care is "the aspect of humanity that refers to the way individuals seek and express meaning and purpose and the way they experience their connectedness to the moment, to self, to others, to nature and to the significant or sacred" (Pulchalski et al., 2009,

p. 887). A cautionary note about the term *spirituality*: Hospice is concerned with bringing people together at the end of life, not with debating semantics or worldviews. Spirituality is not a word most atheists use. When a hospice staff member uses the word in reference to a nonbeliever, clarity of purpose would be helpful to understand how it is used. Staff members in your organization may need additional education on the clear distinction between the inherent spirituality of each person and the related, but separate, religious belief each may have. Historically, there has been confusion with the word *spirituality* (Mais, 2010), and its use can lead to failure in establishing a caring relationship between providers and patients. I ask readers to consider why *spirituality* is used in communication with or about patients who do not adhere to a belief in God. The consensus definition of spirituality is clear and does not assume a belief in a god and is used to frame this chapter.

Having issued caution on the use of the word, it is important to examine the motivation to provide hospice care within generally accepted guidelines and standards.

The imperative to provide spiritual care to atheists is rooted in a desire to serve people at the end of life and to follow professional guidelines. The National Consensus Project Guidelines describes eight domains of care. Spiritual care is the fifth domain: "Spiritual and existential dimensions are assessed and responded to based on the best available evidence, which is skillfully and systematically applied" (Puchalski et al., 2009). Each aspect of the spiritual care of atheists will be described below. Each of the four preferred practices described by the National Consensus Project Guidelines will be reviewed with a discussion of how each relates to atheists.

20: Develop and document a plan based on an assessment of religious, spiritual, and existential concerns using a structured instrument and integrate the information obtained from the assessment into the palliative care plan.

Assessing patients and family members for admission to palliative care and hospice care involves a comprehensive set of questions. One of the most common questions is, "What is your religion?" I suggest this question be changed to, "What is your religion, if any?" Modification of the question allows the patient to know that possessing a religion is not an expectation. Once the patient's belief system is clarified, a more comprehensive analysis of the family's belief system is necessary. The patient and family needs are identified separately. Hodge (2005), a social worker, has described the use of spiritual *ecomaps* as a useful tool to understand the diversity and complexity of the individual philosophies within a family. The spiritual ecomap for my family is presented in Figure 1. Elsewhere in this book are references to other spiritual assessment tools. Agencies should select a tool based on their agency location and community needs.

FIGURE 1. Modified Spiritual Ecomap for the Smith-Stoner Family

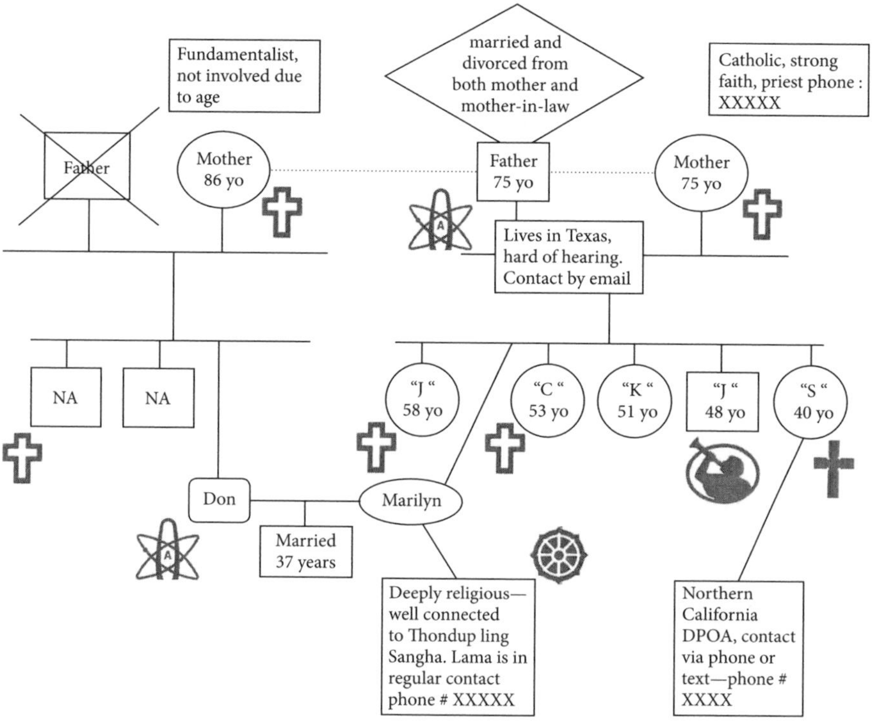

Interventions can be identified by deconstructing the definition of spirituality into three broad groups. First, the way individuals seek and express meaning and purpose to self; second, connectedness to others; and third, connectedness to nature or the significant.

Interventions to address the meaning and purpose of the *self* for atheists are well known to healthcare workers. They should focus on reaffirming life accomplishments, offering and giving forgiveness, life review, and rejoicing in good deeds, as well as related interventions.

The second group of spiritual needs focus on connectedness to others. Being with family and friends, making new friends, and building relationships are important, life-affirming interventions. Using humor can be a welcome method of communication and connection. If some members of the patient's family have religious faith, a chaplain may be appropriate to assure them that they have the support they need. Obtaining such support is a loving act that helps reinforce the desire to remain connected to family members through death.

Finally, connection to nature or the significant suggests that healthcare workers provide opportunities to experience the outdoors. Pets, plants, and anything alive are meaningful additions to the life of a nonbeliever. Concerns about the natural world are also a part of postmortem plans. Most atheists will want to be cremated, using the least amount of resources necessary.

21: Provide information about the availability of spiritual care services and make spiritual care available either through organizational spiritual care counseling or through the patient's own clergy relationships.

The importance of protecting patients from unwanted and unsolicited contact by informal or formal religious representatives who haphazardly share their beliefs about an afterlife cannot be overstated. Atheists in my study, and in many conversations, share a belief that there is no existence after death. Using this information, care should be patient-centered—in other words, secular. Spiritual care includes secular rituals and activities focused on supporting patient-specific goals. Typically, this means ensuring that the patient has time to reflect on life and identify important activities not yet accomplished. Other spiritual care includes affirming or repairing meaningful relationships with friends and family and nurturing the patient's connection to the natural world.

Silence, meditation, and sharing personal stories of life events are the focus of these secular rituals. Reading poetry, listening to music, experiencing the outside world, spending time with family, and recording memories in multiple ways—these are the heart of all spiritual care.

When rituals are performed, especially after death, symbols of nonbelief should be honored and respected by all interdisciplinary team members. The symbol for Atheist grave markers is an atom with the bottom orbit open.

When a patient exhibits symptoms of an existential crisis, the psychological support team should provide appropriate follow-up. An existential crisis is a psychological crisis that requires intervention by the interdisciplinary team. Patients suffering from overwhelming feelings of loneliness or hopelessness require skilled intervention by team members trained in crisis management. Suggestions for supporting an existential crisis include helping patients find meaning in their lives. Important interventions include forgiveness (of self and others) and reconciliation (Worthington, 2006). Many patients fear death and experience hopelessness and despair. As their bodies change and their functional capacity decreases, they experience a variety of emotional reactions. Social workers, counselors, nurses, and physicians all have a role in assisting patients and families adjust to the patient's changing physical condition. Documentation of patient-specific interventions for each discipline is maintained in the plan of care and patient record. All members of the team should be working as one to accomplish a peaceful death.

An interesting alternative view of the use of a chaplain in end-of-life care is presented by Lisa Mais (2010), a former intensive care nurse who now works as a hospice nurse. She describes several reasons for including a chaplain in the care team. The most important is his or her emotional support for a patient and family and his or her ability to plan for memorial care after the patient's death.

22: Specialized palliative and hospice care teams should include spiritual care professionals appropriately trained and certified in palliative care.

The primary objection of atheists is the emphasis given to a chaplain as the sole expert in spiritual matters. Several other palliative care professionals are able to provide highly skilled support for atheists and their families (see Appendix). They include psychologists, social workers, and marriage and family counselors. For atheist families, I suggest that social workers provide the primary spiritual care, focused on helping patients identify the meaning in their own lives, affirm or repair their connection to family members, and assist with life-completion tasks. Their education and experience qualify them to provide this type of care. When more is needed, additional psychological care professionals can be included in the plan of care.

What Is It That Atheists Want from Us?

Without exception, atheists want evidenced-based healthcare that optimizes their function as long as it is effective. They want healthcare workers who are experts in the science of medicine, psychology, social work, nursing, and related professions. Atheists want care providers working with the interdisciplinary care team to reinforce patient autonomy and keep them informed of all relevant information. In other words, atheists want what we all want.

They generally do not want referrals and recommendations for many complementary treatments now common in hospice. These may include the use of energy medicine such as Reiki and therapeutic touch. Many will question healthcare providers on the scientific evidence for any nontraditional medical care recommendations.

Patients who are nonbelievers want our help to stay connected to loved ones as long as quality of life exists. This often means family members will need some coaching. There are an unlimited number of important books on communicating with people who are dying. Two I have found to be very effective are Halpern's *The Etiquette of Illness* (2004) and Byock's *The Four Things That Matter Most* (2004).

The need to forgive and be forgiven is a common concern at the end of life. Byock and many other experts emphasize the significance of forgiveness at the end of life. Luskin (2002) provides an explanation of the science of forgiveness. The clear presentation of the benefits from (and evidence for) positive outcomes related to forgiveness provides important information for patients and their family members.

AFTER-DEATH CARE

One of the most common fears of atheist colleagues, patients, and family is that an after-death religious representative will conduct a memorial service based on religious tradition. Organizing or participating in such a service would be the ultimate breach of professional duty. The plan of care for all patients continues until the end of contact with the family, which includes after death. The patient's wishes must be honored in death just as in life.

However, hospice care is family-centered care. Many families are diverse in their worldviews. If members of a family are requesting comfort from readings in the Bible, consider the passage read by Christopher Hitchens, noted atheist, at his father's funeral:

> *Finally, brethren, whatsoever things are true, whatsoever things are honest, whatsoever things are just, whatsoever things are pure, whatsoever things are lovely, whatsoever things are of good report: If there be any virtue, and if there be any praise, think on these things.* (Philippians 4:8, quoted in Hitchens, 2007a, p. 12)

A simple prayer with grieving families members meant to comfort may be appropriate. Healthcare team members can clarify this with the patient.

Allowing them to see the passages shared with family would be an important intervention to support the patient's autonomy. There is a lot of information on secular funerals. For a funeral, Epstein (2009) suggests the following rituals for nonbelievers:

1. Share stories, laugh, remember, cry.
2. Read from poetry, literature.
3. Tell mourners the person's life story, in photos, in anecdotes, and in mementos.
4. Allow time for silent presence.
5. Quoting from Jane Wilson's funeral guidebook for atheists (1991): *We now come to the final moment of the physical existence of X, with respect, honour, affection, regard and love. His passion and intelligence we commit to our memories. His humanity and caring we commit to our hearts. His body we commit to be burned and returned the cycles of nature he understood so well. "Earth to earth, dust to dust, ashes to ashes."*

LAST WORDS ON ATHEIST COLLEAGUES

A discussion of atheist patients is not complete without a discussion of the experiences of nonbeliever staff members. Without exception, their comments mirror the experiences of patients. I have heard hundreds of stories of frustration from nonbeliever staff members working in an organization that responds primarily to the needs of religious employees. When every staff meeting begins with a theist ritual, there is a lack of sensitivity to the diversity of hospice professionals. My suggestion is simple: Do an organizational assessment. Do not assume that everyone who wears a cross is a believer. Ask staff members how they feel about the rituals provided at meetings.

When I started my work researching atheist preferences for end-of-life care, a colleague expressed her appreciation to me for giving a voice to atheists. Like many others, she told me about her experiences being an atheist in what she described as a largely Christian nursing profession. I was curious because she always wore a simple gold cross around her neck. As far as I could remember, she had it on every day. As my eyes focused on the cross, she simply said, "This cross was my mother's…I loved my mother. I wear it in her memory." I had made many assumptions about the worldview of this dear colleague based simply on one data point—a piece of jewelry.

During your next staff meeting, do a spiritual assessment with the staff. You are likely to discover some atheists in the group. Talk to them and then evaluate their inclusiveness of your organization. Make a commitment to honor the beliefs of all patients *and* staff in personally meaningful, secular ways. Consider how meetings begin and end and how everyone may feel included.

An effective tool for starting a discussion on end-of-life care, and all the emotions included in the process of dying, from a secular point of view is reading *Chapter 12: After You Die* in the Ricky Gervais dark comedy, *The Invention of Lying*. In this fictitious world, no one knows how to lie, until Gervais's character discovers he can lie. As his mother reaches the end of her life, she is in a classic existential crisis, feeling alone and afraid to die. She tells her son she is afraid to die, "…an eternity of nothingness. …I am afraid". Her son responds with a beautiful description of life after death: an existence not previously described in this rational world. Describing a life after death where there is only love, the town is turned into chaos as everyone wants to know more about the previously unknown life after death. Staff may find viewing some or all of the movie as very helpful in starting a conversation about caring for nonbelievers and what constitutes appropriate intervention.

23: Specialized palliative and hospice spiritual care professionals should build partnerships with community clergy and provide education and counseling related to end-of-life care.

Hospice professionals will find no shortage of atheist groups in their community. Ask representatives to come to your hospice and provide education. If none are readily available, there are many groups online. Developing a standard of care for patients who are atheists will be very helpful for staff to understand the importance of maintaining professional boundaries while providing patient-centered care. Additional education will also help clarify the difference between the secular aspects of spirituality and the extended definition, which includes religious dogma. Some staff may feel a great deal of intrapersonal distress in caring for someone who does not belong to a religious tradition. Flexibility in assigning patients to clinicians experiencing their own distress in this situation would help both the staff members and patient. An analogy may be helpful to discuss with staff who feel a deep sense of need to promote a religious conversion in their patient care. If a patient has an allergy to penicillin, it would be considered malpractice to decide that the allergy does not exist and administer penicillin for an infection. The same is true of the belief system for an atheist. Their world view based on nonbelief cannot be discarded just as an allergy warning cannot be discarded by the healthcare team.

Reaching out to members of the local atheist community will help organizations develop patient-centered care guidelines and provide the necessary community linkages to provide authentic, patient-centered care. Creating partnerships with nonbelievers will add to the ability of palliative care professionals to serve more patients and their families.

Marilyn Smith-Stoner, RN-BC, PhD, *has been working in end-of-life care since 1992. As a nursing educator, she works with nursing students and travels internationally to consult with others in China, Brazil, Thailand, the Gambia, and other countries. The needs of diverse individuals: Buddhists, atheists, and Wiccans are among some of the groups she has studied. She is currently focused on developing her concept of the "Silver Hour," which is the metaphorical 30 minutes before and after death. Her goal is to transform the death experience of patients and their families members whenever and where the death occurs. Using the Silver Hour, prehospital, hospital, and home care healthcare workers can focus their care to provide a patient-centered premortem and family-centered post-mortem experience. Two individuals inspire Dr. Smith-Stoner to continue work in developing skill and insight into the care needs of people at the time of and after death. The first is Teresa Ferrara, her great-grandmother, one of the first female Italian embalmers in the United States. The most important influence in her life is the Venerable Lama Chödak Gyatso Nubpa, the most loving and caring person, who died in 2009.*

APPENDIX: RESPONSE TO MY COLLEAGUES IN REVIEWING THE SPIRITUAL CARE GUIDELINES

In discussions with atheist colleagues and upon sharing the consensus definition of *spirituality* with them, Tom Flynn, the editor of the *Skeptical Inquirer*, offers a representative response:

> I looked over the new spirituality guidelines. While much of it is unexceptionable, I did notice some red flags. In its early sections, the paper seems to treat spirituality as a balloon term whose swollen meaning encompasses aspects of care that might better be approached as emotional, affective, or psychological. Thereafter, spirituality is treated more conventionally, as a slightly more-inclusive synonym for religious. I saw no explicit recognition that the outcome of a spirituality inventory could be

that a given patient who was wholly nonspiritual, though I note with approval that there was no language of the sort one so often sees to the effect that "everyone is spiritual whether they think they are, or not." Still, the end result is that the guidelines offer no guidance to the practitioner whose patient denies all interest in things spiritual. Finally, in its closing recommendations, the guidelines seem too narrowly focused on assigning the spiritual care of all patients to pastoral personnel. Though I spotted a lone mention of therapists, I think the issue of nonspiritual patients who disdain all pastoral care and would prefer a psychotherapist or psychologist as their first responder for emotional care is unfortunately omitted.

REFERENCES

Byock, I. (2004). *The four things that matter most: A book about living.* New York: Free Press.

Epstein, G. M. (2009). *Good without God: What a billion nonreligious people do believe.* New York: HarperCollins.

Halpern, S. (2004). *The etiquette of illness: What to say when you can't find the words.* New York: Bloomsbury.

Hitchens, C. (2007a). *God is not great: How religion poisons everything.* New York: Hatchette Book Group.

Hodge, D. R. (2005). Developing a spiritual assessment toolbox: A discussion of strengths and limitations of five different assessment methods. *Health and Social Work, 30*(4), 314–323.

Luskin, F. (2002). *Forgive for good.* San Francisco: Harper.

Mais, L. (2010, Jan–Feb). Perspectives on death and dying from an atheist nurse. *Austin Atheist, 3*(1), 1–4.

National Consensus Project for Quality Palliative Care (2009). *Clinical Practice Guidelines for Quality Palliative Care,* (2nd ed.). Available from www.nationalconsensusproject.org

Oxford Dictionary. (2010). Oxford University Press. Available from www.oxforddictionaries.com

Puchlaski, C., Ferrell, B., Virani, R., Otis-Green, S., Baird, P., Bull, J.,… Sulmasy, D. (2009). Improving the quality of spiritual care as a dimension of palliative care: The report of the consensus conference. *Journal of Palliative Medicine, 12*(10), doi:10.1089/jpm2009.0142.

Smith-Stoner, M. (2007). End-of-life preferences for atheists. *Journal of Palliative Medicine, 10*(4), 923–8.

Worthington, E. (2006). *Forgiveness and reconciliation: Theory and application.* New York: Routledge.

Wilson, J. W. (1991). *Funerals without God: A practical guide to nonreligious funerals.* New York: Prometheus Books.

CHAPTER 17

New Age and Old Age Spiritualities: End-of-Life Care for Wiccans, Pagans, and Nature Spiritualists

Marilyn Smith-Stoner

N ew Age and Wiccan spirituality share many common themes. New Age beliefs are a combination of traditional spiritual practices and Wiccan, Pagan, and newer beliefs, such as the power of dreams. Describing the two belief systems together will help the reader understand that, like others, spiritual worldviews are fluid and some have boundaries that are not well defined. Key to understanding both the New Age beliefs and what some might call *old age beliefs* is that these are decentralized, flexible, and often applied in an individual's life in a highly individualized way. There is no one identifiable book or person that speaks for any of the belief systems. What is presented in this chapter is based on interviews, readings, and experiences derived from participant observations. A description of each of the beliefs will be presented using key parts of the National Consensus Project definition of spirituality: expression of meaning and purpose and connectedness to the moment, to self, to others, and to the significant or sacred (Puchalski et al., 2009).

Other similarities between these two and other religions:

- Strong sense of personal responsibility for life events
- May take on a spiritual name, either given to them or selected. Some may want to be called by this name, even if it is not the legal name
- Death is a transition, and is not the end of existence
- Optimistic attitude toward life and death
- Belief in the healing power of intention, foods, herbal supplements, and many other therapies

- Relationship with spiritual beings: angels, guides, departed loved ones, including animals
- Wide use of symbols, often highly personalized
- Focus on the Goddess and the feminine
- Reverence for the natural world as embodied in Nature, Gaia, or Mother Earth
- Interconnectedness of Earth, people, animals, and the life after death
- An appreciation of beauty, most notably Mother Earth, but including music, poetry, art, and literature

NEW AGE

The term *New Age* was first used as early as 1809 by William Blake, who described a belief in a spiritual and artistic New Age in his preface to *Milton*. Blake describes "Oh Young Men of the New Age..." (p. 95). According to the Religious Tolerance website, the New Age Movement is a "free-flowing spiritual movement" (Religious Tolerance, n.d.). A comprehensive history of New Age spirituality can be found in: *The New Age: The History of a Movement* by Nevill Drury (2004).

The first and foremost of New Age beliefs is the emphasis on an individual's ability to impact this and future lives. Positive thinking in order to create one's own reality, intentional actions, and constant interaction with individuals such as relatives, angels, and spirit guides are a dominant belief across New Age publications. New Age believers, like other religious group members, are in constant interaction with people who have lived and died. Some of the beings who have died are called spirits, others angels, and sometimes guides. These beings are real, and mostly exert a positive influence, including an ability to influence life events. Encouraging a person who is coming to the end of life to contact spiritual partners may bring significant relief from suffering. Identifying those spirits by name and incorporating them into the plan of care contributes to quality patient-centered care.

Death is usually seen as a transition to another world, and New Agers often use the term "heaven." Nearly all authors of New Age publications view the afterlife as positive. Death is a transition—a normal process. Believers will often incorporate a wide range of traditional and complementary therapies into their lifelong health practices. Spiritually sensitive care means healthcare workers honor these requests and negotiate the plan of care with knowledge of potential side effects and interactions of mixing foods, herbal supplements, and prescription medication.

HEALTH BELIEFS

A view of health as holistic is a foundational belief. There is no possible separation of body, mind, and spirit. Health beliefs of New Age people go beyond traditional evidenced-based health care. Many New Age practitioners complement—and sometimes substitute—traditional care with a variety of beliefs and practices. The most commonly mentioned beliefs relevant to end-of-life care are a focus on food as a therapeutic intervention, herbal supplementation, extensive use of energy medicines (Reiki, therapeutic touch, and aromatherapy, among others), and use of all types of alternative practitioners.

HEALTHCARE WORKERS

The healthcare team will likely include practitioners of many alternative healing systems. Asking about and inviting these practitioners into team meetings is not only patient-centered, but is also necessary for patient safety. Understanding the impact of herbal supplements and ritual activity will assist the healthcare team to adjust the plan of care, especially medications.

Concepts such as reading auras or external energy fields may be an issue for some patients. Specially trained aura readers who can see the multicolored light field that surrounds the body may have some influence in diagnosing mental or physical states of both the patient and people who are present in the area with the patient. Although an ethical standard of asking permission for such a reading exists, such diagnoses can have a powerful influence on the patient and family.

Reverence for Earth is especially important when disposable medical equipment is used and disposal of medications and other supplies happen. Some of the most significant spiritual pain and suffering can inadvertently come from not clarifying and negotiating the use of disposable supplies and in the removal of equipment and medications.

Hospice workers strengthen a patient and family when they address the patient's connection to self, connection to others, and connection to the significant or sacred, which includes Mother Nature. Each aspect of the national consensus definition of spirituality will be considered independently.

CONNECTEDNESS TO SELF

A focus on interpersonal issues is vital. This includes support for autonomy in patient decision-making, especially in medication and treatment schedules; addressing the common emotions of grief, sadness, and the desire for transcendence; the need to offer and receive forgiveness; giving and receiving love; and preserving dignity. These are critical to patient-centered care. Many New Age practitioners will see acceptance of their use of health practices that are not scientifically evidenced-based as affirmation of them as individuals.

Life review, journaling, and other ways to document the past are all effective methods of supporting intrapersonal connection to self. Healthcare practices believed to strengthen the self include meditation, guided imagery, prayer, massage, yoga, healing rituals with crystals, predicting life events through horoscopes or Tarot cards, and reading of auras or energy fields.

The benefits of guided imagery and meditation for stress relief and symptom management are well known. Meditation and breathing exercises are part of a long lineage of health and religious practices. Specific research in the benefits of meditation, including breathing exercises and ecospiritualism, is starting to emerge (Delaney & Barrere, 2009). Strengthening a patient's coping with the many changes that typically accompany death is critical to quality care. The positive benefits are increased when interventions are tailored to meet the specific philosophy of the patient.

Combining breathing and meditation with guided imagery, which is often thought of as a meditation, helps to support the death transition. A search on YouTube (www.youtube.com) will identify many examples of New Age-appropriate guided imagery activities. One practitioner to consider is Belleruth Naparstek. Metaphors are important in spiritually specific guided imagery. Terms such as energy, love, light, and angels would be suitable for use. Noting terms that the patient and family use is helpful to incorporate into guided imagery.

Prayer may take many forms and may include a wide array of wishes, aspirations, and requests. Many times, prayers include mention of the ultimate source of life, often a feminine being. Silence is also a commonly accepted form of prayer that incorporates meditation and breathing.

Massage has been found helpful in a wide variety of conditions. Many types of massage can provide benefit for all patients at end of life (Hillier, Louw, Morris, Uwimana, & Statham, 2010). Use of massage therapists is increasingly common in palliative care. Some may have expertise in other energy therapies, such as Reiki (traditional form of Japanese and Tibetan healing). Patients with a New Age spiritual preference will look to complementary practitioners, especially practitioners of therapies such as massage, as massage affirms their beliefs holistically.

Crystals are minerals believed to have healing powers. By breaking down the forces behind illness and injury, a therapeutic effect is thought to be achieved. Crystals are usually combined with the other health practices discussed here, especially breathing and guided imagery. Many homes will have an altar with sacred symbols and crystals displayed. Jewelry made of crystal, especially pieces designated to be cremated with the patient, may also be worn.

Horoscopes and Tarot are individualized methods of understanding forces that impact life events. Using specific data on the time and location of a birth, astrologers can utilize the location of planets and other objects in the sky to predict and explain events. Sometimes horoscopes are referred to as divinations, similar to Buddhist beliefs in the ability to predict future events. Tarot cards are usually decks of 78 cards with various themes associated with mysticism. Experienced Tarot card readers can provide readings of the Tarot locally or over a distance. Asking patients about any readings they have had (horoscope, Tarot, or others) can be helpful in understanding their worldview and what unseen forces they feel are active in their lives. Many of the readings are very detailed and prescriptive. They go well beyond the simple horoscopes in the newspaper. As such, they are a potent influence in the lives of patients.

Dreams are powerful methods of connecting with the afterlife and in translating events on Earth. Asking about dreams gives important insight into the patient experience. Asking the patient to interpret the dream, including images that may be thought of as nearing-death experiences, helps build trust.

CONNECTEDNESS TO OTHERS

Maintaining connection with loved ones is the second core value of spiritual care. Helping patients stay connected and reconnect with friends and family provides the patient with some of the most profound healing at the end of life. The sense of being a burden and coping with the loss of self is as common in people of the New Age and traditional Wiccan beliefs as in other people. Helping family members balance the demands of caregiving strengthens spiritual connections.

The seamless connection with those who are living and dead is central to the New Age philosophy. Remaining connected, including receiving direction on activities in life, is a source of support and encouragement. In addition to conversations and prayers directed at those who have died, there are some specific practices in which a person can have a direct connection. One common practice is to seek out an expert who can channel or communicate directly with those who are dead.

Channeling is a process of communicating with people who have died through another person who channels their spirits and becomes their earthly voice. Some patients may be comforted by seeking out someone who is a channeler of people who have died to ask about the process. The most famous being believed to have been channeled is Seth, who was channeled by Jane Roberts and who dictated many popular books with his wisdom. An Internet search will identify many people who are channelers and many printed resources.

CONNECTEDNESS TO THE SIGNIFICANT OR SACRED

The identification of the sacred for many New Age practitioners often includes a view that all life comes from a single divine source. There is a deep connection to Earth, Mother Nature, Gods, and Goddesses; their spirits are an integral part of human existence. New Age believers are deeply connected to Earth and committed to preserving and enhancing the ecosystem of the planet, which is often referred to as Gaia.

Reincarnation is generally accepted and some believe they made a deliberate choice of who their parents were and the time and place they were born. The sense of being reborn is comforting and fosters the sense of sacredness of dying.

There is a general belief that all religions are one. Incorporation of beliefs from all religions is generally seen as positive, as long as the belief is not mutually exclusive or negatively judges or excludes other beliefs, for example, a monotheist belief in one God. The sacred may be referred to as the *Light*, which refers to the essence of life.

NATIVE AMERICAN SPIRITUALITY

Many New Age practices combine a variety of traditional practices. Native American rituals are popular and incorporated by native and nonnative Americans into their spiritual and religious practices. Palliative care workers may consider incorporating Native American rituals into their multicultural spiritual practices. However benevolent that desire may be, there is another aspect to simply taking another set of practices into one's own portfolio of skills. Four chiefs of Native American tribes asked non-Indians to refrain from doing this at the Parliament of World Religions held in Chicago in 1993, which was the 100th anniversary of the first Parliament of World Religions. Listening to the Native Americans who spoke, as they urged the crowd to not utilize their rituals in non-Indian spiritual events, was one of the most touching moments I have experienced. An example of their sentiments is described in the "Declaration of War against the Theft of Lakota Spirituality" (Lakota, Dakota and Nakota Nations, 1993). The Lakota demand to refrain from using their rituals is significant, and adherence to their requests a part of professional practice.

WICCANS, PAGANS, AND NATURE SPIRITUALISTS

> *I am Pagan. I honor the seasons of life within my life's journey—beginnings, growth, fruition, harvest, endings, rest, and beginnings again. Life is a Circle with many cycles. With every Ending comes a new Beginning. Within Death there is the promise of Rebirth.*
> —Selena Fox (Senior High Priestess, Circle Sanctuary)

Wiccan, Pagans, and Nature Spiritualists (WPNS) have continued to gain popularity in the United States since the publication of "Spiritual Needs of Wiccan, Pagan, and Nature Spiritualists at End of Life" (Smith-Stoner & Young, 2007). WPNS represent a set of common values that are practiced by individuals who may or may not have a direct religious representative guiding their spiritual practice. Practice is more informal and personalized when it takes place in small groups and often outside in places with special meaning during specific times of the year, such as the equinox and solstice. Their symbol for the most important elements is the pentagram.

Wicca and related beliefs continue to be popular (Cush, 2007). Potentially 50% of WPNS practice on their own and may rely on hospice professionals to provide the primary source of religious support when they are unable to perform their own rituals. Wiccan beliefs are popular with teenagers, most recently the subject of a popular series of teen books, *Circle of Three,* in which stories of spiritual growth are mixed into teen witch stories with positive representations of their bodies and common moral dilemmas faced by young adults (Jarvis, 2008).

In a 2006 online survey conducted by me with the assistance of Nora Cedarwind Young, Wiccan, Pagan, and other practitioners were invited to participate through flyers at appropriate Wiccan conferences and on websites. The response was remarkable, with 2,636 completed surveys obtained. The findings presented in Table 1 represent a portion of the results. To summarize the results, the plurality of the participants was 36–50 years old (44%) and lived in the central part of the United States (26%). Along with those living in the northeast (22%), this accounted for nearly half of the responses.

When asked to describe the term they use for their religion, *Pagan* is the preferred term for 32%, and *Wiccan* for 27%, while nearly half (45%) of the participants used other terms. Some of the terms used included *Heathen*, *Animist*, *Asatru*, and *Druid*. A large number of participants had been practitioners for at least 5 years (24%).

TABLE 1. 2006 Online Survey Responses n= 2,636

Selected items		Results	
Age	18–35 years	862	(33%)
	36–50 years	1157	(44%)
	51–65 years	568	(22%)
	66 or older	43	(2%)
Location	Northwest	289	(11%)
	Central	678	(26%)
	Northeast	577	(22%)
	Southeast	424	(16%)
	Other	358	(14%)
Term used to describe religion	Wiccan	723	(27%)
	Pagan	837	(32%)
	Nature Spirituality	297	(11%)
	Combination/other	1151	(45%)
Length of time practicing religion	<5 years	511	(19%)
	5–10 years	644	(24%)
	10–15 years	577	(22%)
	>15 years	877	(33%)
Advance directive completion	Yes	779	(30%)
	No	1828	(70%)
Have shared end-of-life preferences with family	Yes	2191	(83%)
	No	443	(17%)

TABLE 1. *(continued)*

Selected items		Results	
End-of-life preferences include	Feeding tube	241	(9%)
	Breathing machines	264	(10%)
	Narcotic pain medication	1867	(71%)
	Experimental treatments/ surgery	609	(23%)
	Death at home	1748	(67%)
	Cremation	1969	(75%)
	Donation of organs	1776	(68%)
Uses a magical name in faith-related practices	No name	852	(32%)
	Used on in the context of religion	1015	(39%)
	Yes—all the time	765	(29%)
Belief in reincarnation	Do not believe in reincarnation	120	(5%)
	Reincarnation human to human	1076	(41%)
	Reincarnation between humans and animals	704	(27%)
Regular religious practices	Prayer	1815	(70%)
	Magic	1930	(75%)
	Meditation	2185	(85%)
	Relaxation	2018	(78%)
	Guided Imagery	1560	(60%)
Support physician-assisted suicide	Yes	2136	(82%)
	No	468	(18%)

Regarding issues directly related to end-of-life care, only 30% had completed an advance directive but 83% had discussed their end-of-life preferences with their families, which can be considered an advance directive. Their preferences for end-of-life care are described in Table 1. While Wiccans prefer natural remedies if they are available, 73% want narcotic pain medication if it is necessary. Other strong preferences include a desire for cremation, death at home, and donation of organs if possible.

Perhaps the most notable finding from this study is the 82% who support physician-assisted suicide. As an increasing number of states make physician-assisted suicide legal, practitioners will find more patients asking for this assistance. Asking about the desire to have physician-assisted suicide is important. When patients feel the burden of their disease and want to end their life, there are many appropriate interventions to enhance their comfort. However, the patients may be unaware of the many options available to them.

An increasing number of Pagans utilize a "death midwife" to assist in the dying process. Death midwives are nonlicensed, although often certified in this specialty, and educated in the traditional rituals and practices to assist in the normal process of dying. They help both the patient and family manage the changes associated with death. Their inclusion in the extended interdisciplinary team can provide patient-centered care. Ensuring that after-death rituals are also consistent with a Wiccan belief system continues the bond between healthcare workers and the patient, even in death. Specific days of the year have additional significance. They are listed in Table 2. Since some patients are thought to postpone their deaths until there are personally meaningful days or events, this calendar may be helpful in identifying additional days of special interest to Wiccans.

TABLE 2. Sacred Days in the Wiccan Calendar

Month	Holiday	Symbolism
February 2	Imbolc/Candlemas/Brigid	Dedication
March 20	Ostara/Spring Equinox	Breaking Through
May 1	Beltane/May Eve	Fertility
June 21	Midsummer/Summer Solstice	Sun's Peak
August 2	Lammas/Lughnasadh	First Fruits Harvest
September 22	Mabon/Fall Equinox	Transformation
October 31	Samhain/Hallows Eve	Ancestors/Spirits
December 21	Winter Solstice/Yule	Reflection/Birth of Sun

Assisting with a green burial is a central value for Wiccans. A green burial means no chemicals are used in preparation of the patient's body, the body is cremated, and the cremains are disposed of in Nature. Death midwives can assist with all aspects of perimortem care. A search of the Internet can identify local death midwives. The comprehensive website *The Witches' Voice* (www. witchvox.com) will provide access to a wide range of resources for supporting members of the Wiccan groups of religions.

CONNECTION TO SELF

Adherence to the first rule, called the Wiccan Rede—*Harm none; what you put out returns to you threefold*—is the first step in a life review. Wiccans devote their lives to doing good. This includes living a life based on positive values, contributing to the lives of others, and protecting our Earth and Mother Nature. Interventions to assist them in recalling past and present actions to adhere to this fundamental life-affirming principle are the most important spiritual actions.

At times, patients may indicate a desire to use magic, which is defined as the process of changing consciousness by the use of one's will (Higganbotham & Higganbotham, 2002). Rituals may be used to aid in the management of pain, shortness of breath, or other symptoms. Magic might also be used to ease pain or assist in the passage into the Summerland or Otherland, which is the place where existence continues after death.

WPNS practitioners may be interested in activities that support leaving a legacy to others, especially related to religious practices. Since Pagan religions are passed on through oral traditions, making written or digital recordings of life experiences, religious practices, and final wishes are important. Organ donation, DNA banking for determining inherited diseases in a family, and other offerings would be a spiritual practice and be a way of contributing to their families (Starhawk, 1997). Offering assistance to make a will or a list of where sacred items or tools can be found will help ensure that tools and religious items will not be inappropriately distributed after death.

CONNECTION TO OTHERS

Family and friends, both living and dead, provide support for people at the end of life. Interventions that bring people together, strengthen relationships, and reconnect those who have separated are key to any end-of-life care. Interconnectedness is a dominant theme in Wiccan beliefs (Harwood, 2007).

As previously noted, many practitioners support the dying patient through a specialized role called death midwife. Nora Cedarwind Young is one of a few hospice chaplains who is an ordained priestess and practitioner of Wicca. It is common for Pagans to do rituals and prayers in a circle. When helping a patient, they will often hold hands while surrounding the patient. Community members often join hands and sing, pray, or chant, placing the patient in the center to focus the energy. Many will also practice alternative healing methods such as Reiki, sound healing, massage, and music or color therapy.

CONNECTION TO THE SIGNIFICANT OR SACRED

One of the most dominant features of the Wiccan traditions is the reverence for Nature and all living things. This reverence is especially important in burial practices. An authoritative source for green burial practices is "Ceremonies for Life's Thresholds" (www.thresholdsoflife.org).

The significant or sacred being is often feminine in Wicca. It is a misconception that Wiccans worship Satan. Images of the Earth Mother, including relics, clothing, and jewelry, are likely to be surrounding a Wiccan practitioner. However, there is worship of both a male God and female Goddess in many forms (Berger, Leach, & Shaffer, 2003; Finley, 1991). Identifying the ultimate sources of power and sacred force in the universe will help make care personalized. Descriptions of the significant should be adapted to include vocabulary relevant to WPNS. Worship activities and gatherings are conducted according to the cycles of the seasons and the phases of the moon (Arthur, 2008).

Prayers are important to Wiccans. They can be traditional prayers or personalized to the patient. The following is an example from Nora Cedarwind Young:

> Beloved one, you are dying (dead)
> We are here with you
> Carry with you only love
> May our love carry you
> And show you the way
> We are here with you.

IMPORTANT CONSIDERATIONS

Practitioners of Wicca and related religions often feel discriminated against and are often reluctant to self-identify as members of the religion. This reluctance is especially intense when healthcare workers indicate, directly or indirectly, their adherence to Biblical teachings that denounce Pagans and witches. Talk to staff about their level of comfort with the religious practices of the patient and ensure that all staff will maintain professional boundaries. Sensitivity to the patient and staffing needs may require careful attention to the healthcare workers assigned to patients and family who practice one of the Wiccan faiths. The Wiccan tradition has legal protection as a religion, as a civil right, and in federal courts (WICCA, 1995). The Wiccan symbol of the pentagram is now legally accepted by the federal government to be included on headstones in government graveyards. Pagan religions are a diverse and broad group of beliefs including Wicca, Nature Spiritualists, and Druids. There is a shared set of values and beliefs that is usually a part of the religious systems for practitioners (Starhawk, 1997).

A member of the patient's spiritual path may be able to assist staff with some basic education, or the hospice chaplain may be considered only if this person has had training in the WPNS beliefs and practices. Empathy and professional, ethical care must be assured to all hospice patients. It is necessary to have an environment conducive to practicing rituals, maintaining an altar with sacred items, and a staff open to support patients in their spiritual practices.

Concluding Invitation

This chapter has been an attempt to describe the ancient and the new spiritualities for the interdisciplinary palliative healthcare team. Much of what is included may be new and a cause of concern for those who are new to the ideas or belong to a faith that rejects such beliefs. However, we do not have to believe in the principles of other faiths to be supportive. There are times when the most significant support is awareness of the need to defer the spiritual support to someone else. It is not possible to be an expert in every spiritual philosophy. Even so, it is possible to obtain assistance from a qualified practitioner who can often do as much to support the patient and family through a peaceful death as traditional medical practices. Honoring and strengthening patients' connection to their own visions of what is significant in their lives is sacred palliative care.

References

Arthur, S. (2008). Wicca, the apocalypse and the future of the natural world. *Journal for the Study of Religion, Nature and Culture.* doi: 10.1558/jsrnc. v2i2.199.

Berger, H., Leach, E., & Shaffer, L. (2003). *Voices from the Pagan census: A national survey of witches and neo-Pagans in the United States (studies in comparative religion).* Columbia, SC: University of South Carolina Press.

Blake, W. (1804). *Milton: Preface.* In D. V. Erdman (Ed.), *The complete poetry and prose of William Blake.* Berkeley, CA: University of California Press.

Cush, D. (2007). Consumer witchcraft: Are teenage witches a creation of commercial interests? *Journal of Beliefs and Values.* doi: 10.1080/13617670701251439

Delaney, C., & Barrere, C. (2009). Ecospirituality: The experience of environmental meditation in patients with cardiovascular disease. *Holistic Nursing Practice, 23*(6), 361–369.

Drury, N. (2004). *The new age: The history of a movement.* Australia: Thames & Hudson.

Finley, N. (1991). Political activism and feminist spirituality. *Sociological Analysis, 52*(4), 349–362.

Hillier, S. L., Louw, Q., Morris, L., Uwimana, J., & Statham, S. (2010). Massage therapy for people with HIV/AIDS. *Cochrane Database of Systematic Reviews, 1.* doi: 10.1002/14651858.CD007502.pub2

Harwood, B. (2007). Beyond poetry and magick: The core elements of Wiccan morality. *Journal of Contemporary Religion.* doi: 10.1080/13537900701637528.

Higganbotham, J., & Higganbotham, R. (2002). *Paganism: An introduction to earth-centered religions.* St. Paul, MN: Llewellyn Publishers.

Jarvis, C. (2008). Becoming a woman through Wicca: Witches and Wiccans in contemporary teen fiction. *Children's Literature in Education.* doi: 10.1007/s10583-007-9058-0.

Lakota, Dakota and Nakota Nations. (1993). *Declaration of war against exploiters of Lakota spirituality.* Available at http://puffin.creighton.edu/lakota/war.html

New Age. Retrieved from http://www.religioustolerance.org/newage.htm.

Puchalski, C., Ferrell, B., Virani, R., Otis-Green, S., Baird, P., Bull, J.,… Sulmasy, D. (2009). Improving the quality of spiritual care as a dimension of palliative care: The report of the consensus conference, *Journal of Palliative Medicine, 12*(10), doi:10.1089/jpm2009.0142

Religious Tolerance. (n.d.). *WICCA: A neopagan, earth-centered religion.* Retrieved May 23, 2010 from http://www.religioustolerance.org/witchcra.htm

Smith-Stoner, M., & Young, N, C. (2007). Spiritual needs of Wiccan, pagan and nature spiritualists at end of life. *Journal of Hospice and Palliative Nursing, 9*(5), 279–286.

Starhawk, Nightmare M. (1997).The Reclaiming Collective. *The pagan book of living and dying: practical rituals, prayers, blessings and meditations on crossing over.* San Francisco, CA: HarperSanFrancisco.

Yoga Journal. Yoga Poses. Retrieved August 30, 2010, from http://www.yogajournal.com/poses/finder/browse_categories

Index

A

Abandonment to Divine Providence (de Caussade), 136

ABC News
  poll indicating Americans' belief in an afterlife, 76

Abhedananda, Swami
  Hindu philosophy of death and, 194

Acceptance. *See* Love and acceptance

Achille, M.
  components of spirituality, 8–9

Achterberg, Jeanne
  "healing" definition, 66

Adolescence
  spiritual issues, 23, 25–26
  stages of, 25

Advance directives. *See* Living wills

African Methodist Episcopal Church
  beliefs and practices, 168

Afterlife
  ABC News poll indicating Americans' belief in an afterlife, 76
  Buddhism and, 210–211
  Church of Christ, Scientist and, 148
  Church of Jesus Christ of Latter-Day Saints and, 180
  Hinduism and, 196–198
  Islam and, 182–183
  Jehovah's Witnesses and, 164
  Judaism and, 125–126
  mainline Protestants and, 166
  middle adulthood interest in, 28–29
  New Age spirituality and, 234, 238
  Pentecostal Protestants and, 175

Agnosticism. *See* Atheism

Aisenberg, R.
  reproductive capability and mortality, 27

Alpert, Richard
  Hinduism and, 192

AME Church. *See* African Methodist Episcopal Church

American Association of Colleges of Nursing
  nursing education recommendations, 98

American Baptist Church
  beliefs and practices, 167–168

American Heritage Dictionary
  "ritual" definition, 63

Anabaptist church. *See* Mennonites

Anderson, Megory
  "ritual" description, 64

Anglican church. *See* Episcopal Church in the U.S.

ANH. *See* Artificial nutrition and hydration

Anointing of the Sick
  description, 138–139

Archstone Foundation
  Consensus Project sponsor, 37

Arrien, Angeles
  definition of ritual, 63
  The art and science of reminiscing: Theory, research methods, and applications (Haight and Webster), 79

Artificial nutrition and hydration
  Judaism and, 121
  religious objections and, 58–60

Assemblies of God
  beliefs and practices, 175

Assisted suicide
  Islam and, 189
  Judaism and, 121
  Wiccans, Pagans, and Nature Spiritualists and, 242

Atheism
  after-death care, 227–228
  chaplains and, 225, 226
  community outreach and, 229
  complementary treatments and, 227
  existential crises and, 225–226
  forgiveness and, 227
  hospice staff members and, 221–222
  modified spiritual ecomap for the Smith-Stoner family (figure), 224
  National Consensus Project for Quality Palliative Care guidelines and, 223–226, 229
  protecting patients from unwanted and unsolicited contact with religious representatives, 225
  secular rituals, 225
  social workers for primary spiritual care, 226
  spiritual definition, 222–223
  spiritual ecomaps and, 223–224
  symbol for grave markers, 225
  terminology for, 222
  what atheists want from caregivers, 226–227
  worldview, 222

Aulen, Bishop Gustav
  Christus Victor theory of the Atonement, 151

Aurobindo, Sri
  Hindu philosophy of death and, 194, 195

D

E